Trauma and Pain in Wound Care
volume II

Other titles available from Wounds UK include:

Skin Care in Wound Management: Assessment, prevention and treatment
edited by Richard White

A Pocket Guide to Clinical Decision-making in Wound Management
edited by Sue Bale and David Gray

Paediatric Skin and Wound Care
edited by Richard White and Jacqueline Denyer

Trauma and Pain in Wound Care
edited by Richard White and Keith Harding

Leg Ulcers and Problems of the Lower Limb: An holistic approach
edited by Ellie Lindsay and Richard White

Advances in Wound Care, volume I
edited by Richard White

Honey in Modern Wound Management
edited by Rose Cooper, Peter Molan and Richard White

VAC Therapy: An introduction and practical guide
edited by David Gray, Fiona Russell and John Timmons

Trauma and Pain in Wound Care
volume II

edited by
Richard White and Keith Harding

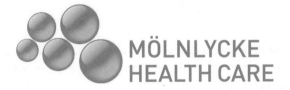

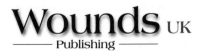

HealthComm UK Limited, trading as Wounds UK Limited, Suite 3.1,
36 Upperkirkgate, Aberdeen AB10 1BA

British Library Cataloguing-in-Publication Data
A catalogue record is available for this book

© HealthComm UK Limited 2009
ISBN-10 0-9555758-4-6
ISBN-13 978-0-9555758-4-6

Printed in Malta by Gutenberg Press Limited, Tarxien, Malta

CONTENTS

CONTRIBUTORS

Hilde Beele is Professor, Department of Dermatology, Ghent University Hospital, Gent, Belgium

Emma Briggs is Lecturer, in Nursing, Department of Acute Adult Nursing, Florence Nightingale School of Nursing and Midwifery, King's College London

Michelle Briggs is Post Doctoral Research Fellow, Leeds Pallium Research Group, School of Healthcare, University of Leeds

Laura Clark is Foundation Year 1 House Officer, Mayday University Hospital, Croydon

Kath Clarke is Lead Nurse Clinical Governance/Practice Development, Wrexham Maelor Hospital, Wrexham

José Contreras-Ruiz, Interdisciplinary Wound and Ostomy Care Centre, 'Dr. Manuel Gea González' General Hospital, Mexico City, Mexico

Jacqueline Denyer is Nurse Consultant for children with epidermolysis bullosa (EB), Great Ormond Street Hospital, London

Hilde Fagervik-Morton is Research Assistant, Department of Wound Healing, School of Medicine, Cardiff University, Cardiff

Patricia Grocott is Reader in Palliative Wound Care, King's College London

Keith Harding is Head of the Department of Wound Healing, School of Medicine, Cardiff University and Clinical Director of Wound Healing in the Cardiff and Vale NHS Trust

Theis Huldt-Nystrøm is Consultant Dermatologist, Hudpoliklinikken i Namsos, Namsos, Norway

Ron Iphofen is Director of Postgraduate Studies, School of Healthcare Sciences, Bangor University, Bangor

Tzvetanka Ivanova-Stoilova is Consultant in Anaesthesia and Pain Medicine, Gwent Healthcare NHS Trust, Royal Gwent Hospital, Newport, Gwent, Wales

Sabu James is Consultant Anaesthetist, Department of Anaesthesia, Monklands Hospital, Airdrie and Lead for Chronic Pain Services, NHS Lanarkshire

Mark Johnson is Professor of Pain and Analgesia, Leeds Metropolitan University, Leeds

Keith Judkins is Consultant Anaesthetist, Mid-Yorkshire Hospitals NHS Trust, Clinical Director, Northern Burn Care Network and Prevention Lead, British Burn Association

Christina Lindholm is Professor of Nursing, Department of Health Sciences, Kristianstad University, Kristianstad, Sweden

Victoria Mason is Lecturer in Applied Psychology, Psychology and Health Sciences, University of Worcester

Sylvie Meaume is Head of Geriatric Department, Hospital Charles-Foix, Ivry sur Seine, France

Britta Melby-Østergaard, RN, Copenhagen Wound Healing Centre, Bispebjerg Hospital, Copenhagen, Denmark

Elizabeth J Mudge is Podiatrist, Department of Wound Healing, School of Medicine, Cardiff University, Cardiff

Yolanda Peter, RN, Fachleiterin Wundbehandlung, Spital Bülach, Bülach, Switzerland

Patricia Price is Professor of Health Sciences, Wound Healing Research Unit, School of Medicine, Cardiff University, Cardiff

Andy Roden is Lecturer, Faculty of Health, University of Wales, Bangor

Marco Romanelli is Director, Wound Healing Research Unit, University of Pisa, Italy

Salla Seppänen is Head of Health Department, Mikkeli University of Applied Sciences, Mikkeli, Finland

Thomas E Serena is Founder and Medical Director of the Penn North Centers for Advanced Wound Care, Warren, PA USA

R Gary Sibbald is Director of Dermatology, Daycare and Wound Healing Clinic, Women's College Hospital, Toronto; Director of the Interdisciplinary Wound Care Course at the University of Toronto

Jose Verdú Soriano, PhD, Department of Community Nursing, Preventive Medicine, Public Health and History of Science, School of Nursing, University of Alicante, Alicante, Spain

Barry Strickland Hodge is Senior Pharmacy Lecturer, School of Healthcare, University of Leeds

Tarnia Taverner is Matron, East Sussex Downs and Weald Primary Care Trust and part-time PhD student, School of Healthcare, University of Leeds

Richard White is Professor of Tissue Viability, Department of Health and Social Care and Psychology, University of Worcester

Wendy White is a Nurse Consultant/Educator (Private Practice), New South Wales, Australia

Uwe Wollina, MD, Allergology & Environmental Medicine, Academic Teaching Hospital of the Technical University of Dresden, Dresden, Germany

Kevin Y Woo is a Clinical Researcher, University of Toronto, Wound Healing Clinic, Women's College Hospital, Toronto, Canada

Carolyn Wyndham-White, RN, HES-Chargée d'enseignement, Geneva, Switzerland

Trudie Young is Lecturer, School of Healthcare Sciences, University of Wales, Bangor

FOREWORD

Since the early 1990s, we have witnessed an ever-increasing interest and level of research activity investigating pain, as it relates to those living with acute or chronic wounds. Early authors and researchers are to be acknowledged for raising the profile of this important practice issue, and for initiating what is today, a growing body of knowledge on the topic. An appreciation of the pathophysiology of wound pain, its multifactorial nature and the profound negative impact on both the person and the wound, has lead to the introduction of the term 'wound-related pain'.

International 'voices' continue to be heard from around the globe and as knowledge increases, so clinical practice is constantly challenged (European Wound Management Association [EWMA], 2002; Reddy *et al*, 2003; World Union of Wound Healing Societies [WUWHS], 2004, 2007). It is recommended that healthcare professionals understand wound-related pain as it affects those individuals in their care, and incorporate a comprehensive initial assessment with ongoing follow-up, including wound-related pain severity scores before, during and after dressing-related procedures.

This text highlights the importance of wound-related pain assessment and provides supportive evidence to assist healthcare professionals in the implementation of individualised pain minimisation strategies (pharmacological and non-pharmacological), and encourage continuous monitoring to identify and address changing individual needs. One could though ask, is wound-related pain assessment 'routine' and how widespread are these practices which aim to understand and improve the individual's experience

This book not only stimulates discussion around these and other wound-related pain questions, but challenges future directions for practice through the dissemination of research findings, including the 'patient's perspective', along with current knowledge/evidence on a range of wound-related pain topics, including the psychology of pain.

As these pages are explored, let us not forget the individuals living and suffering with wound-related pain. Asking 'Could I, my department, my organisation, assess and manage wound-related pain better' is an important question for healthcare professionals, recognising their unique position to impact on the lives of others. When caring for those with acute and chronic wounds, it is the responsibility of healthcare professionals to continually strive to understand and improve the individual's wound-related pain experience.

I recommend this text, as the lives of those in our care can be influenced positively or negatively by our clinical practice, which relates directly to our knowledge and appreciation of wound-related pain.

Wendy White
Nurse Consultant/Educator (Private Practice)
New South Wales
Australia
October, 2008

References

European Wound Management Association (2002) Position Document: *Pain at wound dressing changes*. London: MEP Ltd. Available online at: www.ewma.org

Reddy M, Kohr R, Queen D, Keast D, Sibbald RG (2003) Practical treatment of wound pain and trauma: a patient-centred approach. An overview. *Ostomy Wound Management* 49(4 Suppl): 2–15

World Union of Wound Healing Societies (2004) Principles of best practice: Minimising pain at wound dressing-related procedures. A consensus document. London: MEP Ltd

World Union of Wound Healing Societies (2007) Principles of best practice: Minimising pain at wound dressing-related procedures. A consensus document. Toronto, Ontario, Canada: ©WoundPedia Inc

CHAPTER 1

PHYSIOLOGY OF PAIN

Mark Johnson

The European Wound Management Association (EWMA) Position Document entitled Pain at Wound Dressing Changes acknowledges that pain is a major issue for patients with wounds, and that inadequate treatment of wound pain has been consistently reported (European Wound Management Association Position Document, 2002). Wound pain may be associated with underlying pathology of the wound and/or wound management, such as debridement or dressing changes (Krasner, 1995; Freedman, 2004). An international survey of 11 countries which formed part of the EWMA document, found that patients experience greatest pain during dressing change, and that practitioners rank prevention of pain and wound trauma as the most desired characteristic at a dressing change (Moffatt *et al*, 2002). Interestingly however, practitioners from only two of 11 countries rated giving analgesia as the most important factor before dressing changes (of eight possible options).

Misguided beliefs

Often pain is neglected as a healthcare issue. This may be because people do not die of pain, although many die in pain. Practitioners may give wound pain management a low priority because they are preoccupied with treating visible pathology or they believe that pain is harmless and an unavoidable consequence of having a wound, which is not the case. Some practitioners are fearful of addiction and/ or respiratory depression associated with opioid analgesics (Ready and Edwards, 1992; Cousins and Power 1999). These misguided attitudes can lead to inappropriate pain assessment and insufficient prescribing of analgesia (Scheinfeld, 2005). They often result from insufficient knowledge about the physiology of pain.

Pain is a psychological state. There is no objective way of measuring another person's pain. If a person says they are experiencing pain then they should be believed. Pain generates a state of physiological stress, and this will increase blood pressure, alter blood gases, delay gastric emptying, cause urinary retention, and increase levels of 'stress hormones' such as cortisol (*Figure 1.1*). If pain persists, this physiological stress will be detrimental to the health and healing of a wound. Persistent pain also causes long-term changes in the structure and function of the central nervous system. It is now recognised that many people with chronic pain have a dysfunctional pain system. For this reason, chronic pain should be considered as a disease entity in its own right.

Unfortunately, learning about the physiology of pain is often painful in itself because too much attention is given to physiological minutia. Despite what physiologists may have you believe, practitioners do not need to know the names of all of the molecule substrates that may be

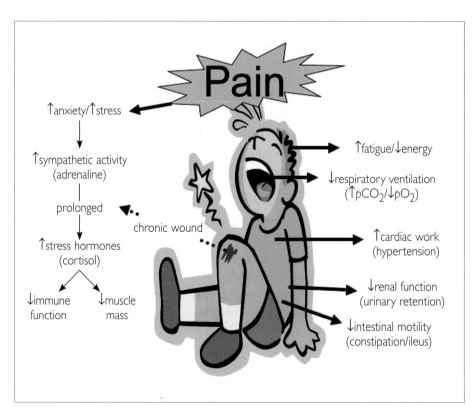

Figure 1.1: Many physiological responses to pain are mediated through the sympathetic division of the autonomic nervous system

involved in pain processing. It is far more important for practitioners to have a working knowledge of the physiological concepts that underpin the types of pain seen in the clinical setting. The purpose of this chapter is to overview the physiological concepts that help in our understanding of pain.

What is pain?

Defining pain

In clinical practice, 'Pain is what the patient says it is' (McCaffery, 1983) and, therefore, related to the person's ability to articulate what they are experiencing. Leg ulceration and superficial burns have been reported to be the most painful wounds with pressure ulcers, cuts, abrasions, and fungating wounds less painful (Moffatt _et al_, 2002; Price _et al_, 2008; _Chapter 2_). However, 'most painful' and 'less painful' are general terms and give little insight to the exact nature of a patient's experience. Patients usually use the term 'pain' in conjunction with adjectives about of the intensity of the pain, the quality of the pain, the extent of the pain, or how bothersome the pain is. These adjectives are crucial in establishing the nature of a patient's pain and are influenced by many factors including type of injury, culture, environment, and individual circumstance (Melzack, 1975; Melzack and Katz, 1999).

The International Association for the Study of Pain (IASP) defines pain as:

> _... an unpleasant sensory and emotional experience associated with actual or potential tissue damage, or described in terms of such damage._
>
> (Merskey and Bogduk, 1994)

This working definition demonstrates that pain is a psychological state and, therefore, a personal experience and always subjective.

The nociceptive system

The body's neural system dedicated to detecting actual or potential tissue damage (i.e. noxious stimuli) is called the nociceptive system and consists of:

3

- *Nociceptors:* Sensory receptor cells preferentially sensitive to noxious stimuli or to stimuli which would become noxious if prolonged (Merskey and Bogduk, 1994).
- *Transmission pathways:* Neural pathways sending nerve impulses from nociceptors to, and within, the central nervous system.
- *Processing areas (perception):* Neural areas in the brain which process incoming impulses to generate an awareness of the noxious stimulus via the sensation of pain (*Figure 1.2*).

However, the IASP definition avoids linking all pain to the presence of tissue damage because the relationship between pain and injury is sometimes very variable.

Pain is difficult to predict

Injury is not always a good predictor of pain, as demonstrated in the following examples:

- an injury may occur without pain, as seen in neuropathic foot ulcers where the reduced sensibility leads to a chronic wound
- an injury may generate pain that is out of proportion to the extent of tissue damage, as seen when a sliver of metal embeds under a finger nail producing excruciating pain
- an injury may have healed yet pain persists, as seen in post-amputation stump pain
- an injury may amplify the intensity of subsequent stimuli, as seen during wound dressings
- an injury may generate pain at a different body location, as seen in referred pain down the arm during a myocardial infarction.

Pain is a multidimensional experience

Pain consists of sensory-discriminative, affective-motivational, and cognitive-evaluative dimensions (Melzack and Katz, 1999; *Figure 1.3*).

- *Sensory-discriminative dimensions* relate to the intensity, location, and quality of the pain, and are sub-served by the nociceptive system and its association with the somatosensory cortex.
- *Affective-motivational dimensions* relate to emotional aspects

of pain and are sub-served by the nociceptive system and its association with the reticular and limbic systems (insula cortex and cingulate gyrus).

- *Cognitive-evaluative dimensions* relate to thoughts and meanings of pain and are sub-served by the nociceptive system and its association with the frontal lobe of the cerebral cortex.

Each dimension of the pain experience must be addressed during treatment and, therefore, a multidisciplinary pain management approach is necessary. Pain of known cause and limited duration, such as minor cuts and abrasions, have modest contributions from affective and cognitive dimensions because the patient expects the pain to disappear as the injury heals. Pain that persists, such as a chronic leg ulcer pain, may have substantial contributions from affective and cognitive dimensions, because the patient does not understand why the wound does not heal.

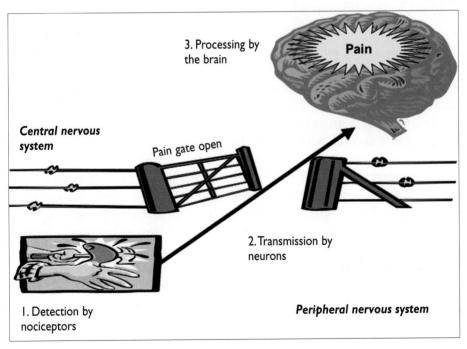

Figure 1.2: Components of the nociceptive system and the 'pain gate'. Activity in the nociceptive neurons opens the 'pain gate' so that impulses can reach higher levels of the brain where they are processed to create a sensation of pain

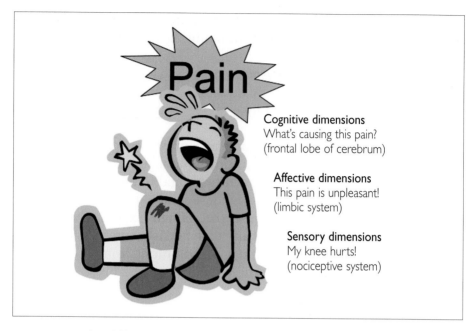

Figure 1.3: The different dimensions of pain

Pain is a dynamic entity

Pain is a dynamic phenomenon that will fluctuate in quality, intensity, and location over time (i.e. seconds, minutes, hours, days, months and years). Wound pain may exist when the patient is resting and in the absence of external stimuli (i.e. background pain). Background pain may persist throughout the day (i.e. static or continuous), or it may be intermittent (episodic). Intermittent pain may be erratic or it may occur in waves and patterns (*Figure 1.4*). There may be a background pain which flares up intermittently from time to time. Wounds are often sensitive to provoking stimuli as occurs during dressing changes or debridement. These provoking stimuli produce particularly intense and distressing pain, which is substantially amplified and out of proportion to the intensity of provoking stimulus.

The nociceptive system can alter its sensitivity

The nociceptive system operates in various states of sensitivity as characterised in *Table 1.1* (Woolf, 1987; Woolf, 1994; Woolf and Salter, 2000; Woolf, 2007).

This is evident if you consider progress of a typical 'household injury', such as a graze or a burn to the skin (*Figure 1.5*).

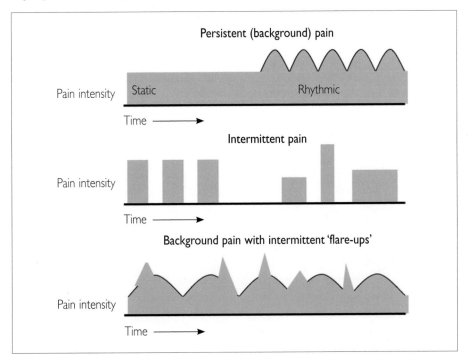

Figure 1.4: Patterns of pain

Pre-injury normal state

The nociceptive system operates in a 'normal state' in healthy individuals who do not have any appreciable tissue damage. In its normal state, the nociceptive system is primed to detect actual or potential tissue damage. When a noxious stimulus occurs, such as spillage of boiling water on to a hand, the nociceptive system will instigate a rapid reflex withdrawal of the body part from the source of the tissue damage. This often occurs before you experience pain (*Figure 1.6*).

A few seconds later, a sharp, intense, localised pain develops (termed first or fast pain) followed by a dull, aching, spreading pain (termed second or slow pain) which is sometimes accompanied by nausea. These two pain sensations result from direct activation of the nociceptive system and their intensity mirrors the intensity of the stimuli. They help us to remember to avoid the stimuli in the future (*Figure 1.6*).

Table 1.1: The characteristics of normal, suppressed and sensitised pain (adapted from Doubell et al, 1999)					
Nociceptive system state	Nociceptive transmission	Peripheral tissue	Afferent input	Sensation	Clinical correlate
Normal (control)	Normal	Healthy	Non-noxious Noxious	No pain Pain	Transient pain
Sensitised	Amplified due to increased excitation or reduced inhibition	Injured	Non-noxious Noxious	Pain (allodynia) Exaggerated pain (hyperalgesia)	Nociceptive and/or neuropathic pain
Persistently sensitised and/ or reorganised	May be amplified or abnormal	May be healthy or injured	Non-noxious Noxious	Pain (allodynia) Exaggerated pain (hyperalgesia)	Persistent nociceptive and/or neuropathic pain
Suppressed	Diminished due to reduced excitation or increased inhibition	Healthy or injured	Non-noxious Noxious	No pain Reduced pain	Pain relief

Suppressed state

The nociceptive system can also operate in a 'suppressed state' whereby the intensity of pain is lower than expected. Pouring cold water over an injury or rubbing the skin close to the injury may provide immediate but short-term pain relief. Reducing pain in this way allows us to continue actions, such as completing an important sporting event, despite the presence of tissue damage. The nociceptive system can also be suppressed by mental distraction and motivational states.

Sensitised state

In healthy tissue, low intensity stimuli produce non-painful sensations, such as touch, hot, cold, and high intensity stimuli produce pain. However, in the presence of tissue damage, low intensity stimuli produce increased pain (allodynia), and high intensity stimuli produce exaggerated pain (hyperalgesia). For example, touching an open wound with your finger produces pain, instead of touch, and pricking an open wound with a needle produces excruciating pain

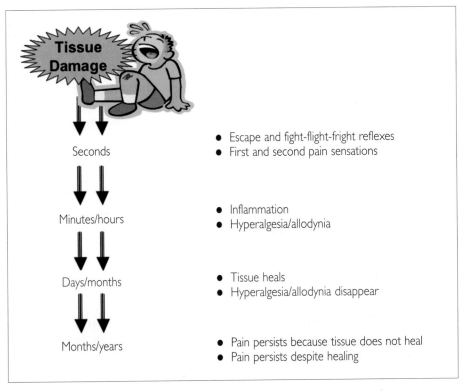

Figure 1.5: Pain-related events following an injury

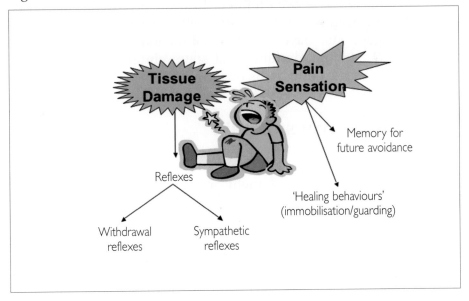

Figure 1.6: Immediate responses to injury when the nociceptive system is operating in its normal pre-injury state

that has a far higher intensity than would be expected for healthy tissue.

In damaged tissue, the nociceptive system operates in a 'sensitised state' to encourage behaviours that guard the injury from further damage and this will aid tissue healing. The sensitised state is recognised by pain in the absence of provoking stimuli (spontaneous pain), tenderness (allodynia), and exaggerated pain (hyperalgesia). Allodynia is, 'pain due to a stimulus which does not normally provoke pain' (Merskey and Bogduk, 1994). Hyperalgesia is, 'an increased response to a stimulus which is normally painful' (Merskey and Bogduk, 1994). Primary hyperalgesia occurs at the site of injury and secondary hyperalgesia occurs in the healthy tissue that surrounds the injury (Merskey and Bogduk, 1994).

Persistently sensitised state — dysfunctional

Normally, the nociceptive system returns to its normal pre-injury state when tissue heals and spontaneous pain, allodynia and hyperalgesia disappear. Sometimes the injury does not heal and the nociceptive system remains sensitised, as seen in some chronic wounds. Sometimes the injury heals but the nociceptive system remains sensitised, as seen when nerves have been injured. In these persistently sensitised states, the nociceptive system may well have developed its own pathophysiology and have become dysfunctional itself (Devor and Seltzer, 1999). In this dysfunctional state, chronic pain should be considered a disease entity in its own right.

Categorising types of pain

Categorisation of pain is fraught with difficulty. Pain has been categorised according to: i) duration (e.g. acute, chronic); ii) cause (e.g. burn, pressure ulcer); iii) anatomical site (e.g. back, headache); iv) system (e.g. visceral, musculoskeletal); and v) physiological mechanism (e.g. nociceptive, neuropathic), to name but a few. Often authors mix category systems in discussions and this has led to confusion in nomenclature and understanding. The most commonly used categorisation of pain in clinical practice is according to the duration of the pain as characterised in *Table 1.2*.

Transient pain (normal state)

Transient pain, sometimes termed phasic pain, is 'pain of brief duration and little consequence....' (Melzack and Wall, 1988; Craig, 2006). It serves to initiate protective responses and to make us aware of stimuli that are damaging so that we can avoid them in the future (*Figure 1.6*, *Table 1.2*).

Acute pain (sensitised state)

Acute pain is 'pain of recent onset and probable limited duration. It usually has an identifiable temporal and causal relationship to injury and disease' (Ready and Edwards, 1992; Merskey and Bogduk, 1994). Acute pain serves to aid tissue repair by making injured areas sensitive to provoking stimuli, as seen during wound dressing changes. Sensations of tenderness (allodynia) and exaggerated pain (hyperalgesia) are often present to promote behaviours that guard and/or immobilise the injured site (*Table 1.2*).

Chronic pain (persistently sensitised state — dysfunctional)

Chronic pain is '....pain lasting for long periods of time' (Ready and Edwards, 1992). Often, 'chronic pain commonly persists beyond the expected time of healing of an injury and frequently there may not be any clearly identifiable cause' (Ready and Edwards, 1992). However, pain may also persist because of ongoing tissue damage as seen in chronic wounds which fail to heal, or in degenerating disease such as arthritis or advanced cancer (Merskey and Bogduk, 1994). Often, chronic pain serves no useful purpose and the nociceptive system itself may have become dysfunctional (*Table 1.2*).

Nociception — the normal pain state

Physiological responses to noxious stimuli

In healthy individuals a noxious stimulus generates a variety of physiological responses.

Table 1.2: The characteristics of transient, acute and chronic pain			
Characteristic	Transient pain	Acute pain	Chronic pain
Provoking stimulus	Noxious causing potential tissue damage	Noxious causing actual tissue damage	Persistent, ongoing tissue damage, or dysfunctional nociceptive system or unknown/other factors
Intensity and time course of pain sensation resulting from stimulus	Related to the severity of stimulus but usually short-lived and of little consequence if tissue damage is minimal	Related to the severity of stimulus and will diminish as tissue heals	May be predictable in the presence of ongoing disease or no relationship between pain and original injury (stimulus)
Status of tissue	Healthy	Damaged	May be healthy or damaged
Response to additional provoking stimuli	Normal Non-noxious stimuli produce non-noxious sensations Noxious stimuli produce pain	Amplified Non-noxious stimuli produce noxious sensations (allodynia) Noxious stimuli produce exaggerated pain (hyperalgesia)	Amplified Non-noxious stimuli produce noxious sensations (allodynia) Noxious stimuli produce exaggerated pain (hyperalgesia)
Physiological symptoms	Nociceptive system activated	Nociceptive system sensitised	Nociceptive system continuously activated by ongoing disease and persistently sensitised
Function	Initiate escape responses to reduce extent of damage Memory of pain-evoking stimuli enables future avoidance	Initiate behaviours that guard/immobilise site of injury to prevent further tissue damage and to promote healing	Initiate behaviours that guard/immobilise site of injury to prevent further tissue damage and to promote healing May be maladaptive — no clear purpose
Semantic correlates	Physiologic pain–nociceptive pain	Nociceptive pain–inflammatory pain	Persistent nociceptive/inflammatory pain Neuropathic pain Pathophysiological pain

Withdrawal (somatic) reflexes

If you pick up something that is 'burning hot' you may well drop it before you experience a sensation of pain. This protective reflex, termed the withdrawal reflex, enables a rapid response to occur without us having to 'think about it'. The withdrawal reflex involves activation of tissue damage receptors (nociceptors), resulting in activity in afferent nociceptive neurons, interneurons in the spinal cord, efferent motor neurons and, ultimately, contraction and relaxation of opposing skeletal muscle groups (_Figure 1.7_).

The neural circuitry involved in the withdrawal reflex is likely to be involved in pains arising in skeletal muscle, such as nocturnal cramps and intermittent claudication associated with arterial disease. It is widely written that the tissue damage can cause persistent skeletal muscle contraction (spasm), leading to a pain-spasm-pain cycle whereby persistent skeletal muscle contraction activates muscle nociceptors and perpetuates a positive feedback loop (_Figure 1.8_). The idea that nociceptor activity causes muscle contraction which, in turn, generates further nociceptor activity causing further contraction has been challenged (Mense and Simons, 2001). Nevertheless, painful muscle spasms will compress blood vessels leading to skeletal muscle ischaemia. It is known that prolonged interruption of the blood supply to the skeletal muscles of resting limbs is not painful in itself. However, pain arises if ischaemic skeletal muscle begins to contract and will

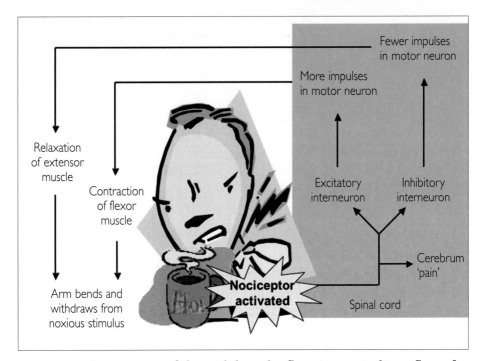

Figure 1.7: Components of the withdrawal reflex. Arrows indicate flow of neural information

increase dramatically with increasing frequency, force, and duration of muscle contraction. These mechanisms are likely to contribute to muscle pains during nocturnal calf cramps seen with chronic venous insufficiency. These mechanisms also contribute to the deep-seated leg pain that occurs when patients with arterial disease walk a predictable distance (i.e. intermittent claudication). These patients find that pain is relieved by a brief rest.

Sympathetic (autonomic) reflexes

Noxious stimuli activate the sympathetic division of the autonomic nervous system (ANS) which releases adrenaline (epinephrine) and noradrenaline (norepinephrine). This causes a fight-flight-fright (stress-like) response and increased blood pressure, leading to hypertension, changes in pulmonary ventilation and alterations in blood gas concentrations, reductions in gastrointestinal motility and constipation, and reductions in bladder emptying and urinary retention (*Figure 1.1*).

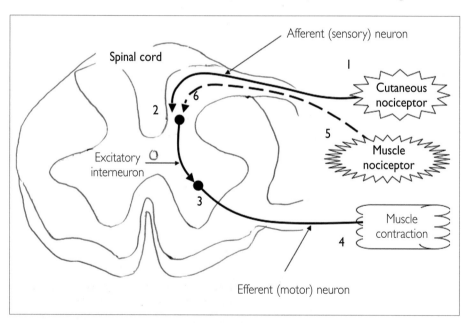

Figure 1.8: Motor reflexes contributing to pain. Activity in nociceptors [1] causes activation of interneurons [2] which, in turn, activate somatic efferent (motor) neurons [3]. Acetylcholine is released at the neuromuscular junction producing an intense and persistent muscle contraction [4] which is detected by muscle nociceptors [5]. The additional afferent information [dashed line] generates further muscle contraction via a positive feedback loop [6]. A positive feedback loop develops

In addition, noxious stimuli cause vasoconstriction in peripheral tissue leading to ischaemia, delayed tissue healing and enhanced nociceptor activity. The release of noradrenaline by sympathetic efferents at the site of tissue damage can sensitise nociceptors with the resultant increase in nociceptor activity forming positive feedback loops which exacerbate pain (*Figure 1.9*). Persistent pain will cause persistent sympathetic activity and an increase in the amount of circulating cortisol, thyroid hormones, and human growth hormone. Cortisol causes muscle wasting, suppression of the immune system, and possible gastrointestinal tract ulceration (Baron and Janig, 2004).

Clearly, the plethora of reflex-induced physiological changes that occur as a result of nociceptor activity are complex and often additive. It is crucial that patients receive pain-relieving interventions to reduce their detrimental impact.

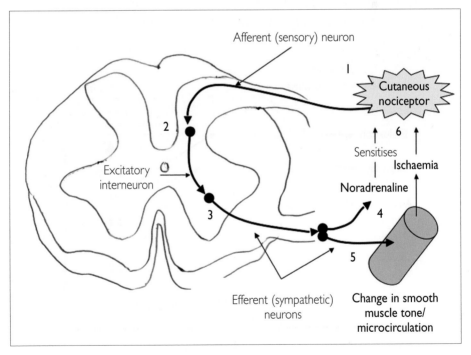

Figure 1.9: Sympathetic reflexes contributing to pain. Activity in nociceptors [1] causes activation of interneurons [2] and pre-ganglionic [3] and post-ganglionic sympathetic neurons. These sympathetic efferents release noradrenaline that sensitises cutaneous nociceptors [4] and causes vasoconstriction in peripheral tissue leading to ischaemia [5], resulting in more activity in nociceptors [6]. A positive feedback loop forms

Psychological responses to noxious stimuli — the sensation of pain

In healthy individuals, a noxious stimulus may become a painful sensation through the processes of transduction, transmission, and perception (*Figures 1.2* and *1.10*).

Transduction

Noxious, or tissue damaging stimuli are detected and converted into nerve impulses by nociceptors in a process called transduction. Nociceptors are, '[sensory] receptor(s) preferentially sensitive to a noxious stimulus or to a stimulus which would become noxious if prolonged' (Merskey and Bogduk, 1994). Nociceptors are 'tissue damage detectors', not 'pain detectors', because the sensation of pain is produced by the brain, not by the receptors. Nociceptors are free nerve endings that respond to high intensity thermal and mechanical stimuli and to chemicals produced by the body following injury

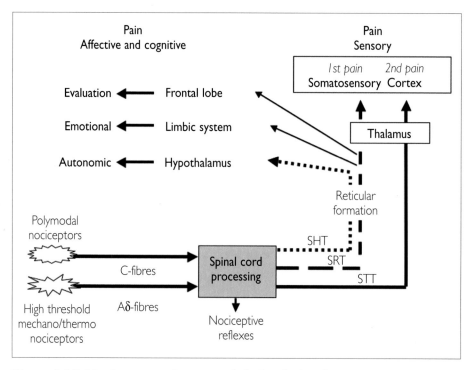

Figure 1.10: Nociceptor pathways and their relationship to sensory, affective and cognitive dimensions of pain. SRT = spinoreticular tract; STT = spinothalamic tract; SHT = spinohypothalamic tract

(*Figure 1.11*) (Raja *et al*, 1999; Basbaum, 2004; Drew and Wood, 2004; Koltzenburg, 2004; Meyer *et al*, 2006).

Nomenclature can be complex and many sub-types of nociceptors have been described. Nociceptors are often classified into:

- *A-fibre nociceptors:* these help to detect stimuli with the potential to damage tissue and respond best to extremes of hot and cold, and to high intensity mechanical events. A-fibre nociceptor activity contributes to reflex responses (e.g. withdrawal reflexes), and to 'first' or 'fast' pain sensations that help to locate the noxious stimuli (e.g. 'pricking' and 'sharp' pain sensations, *Figure 1.10*). A-fibre nociceptors have been sub-classified into type 1 nociceptors, with a predominance of A-fibre mechano-heat nociceptors, and type 2 nociceptors, which are less responsive to mechanical stimuli. Both types of A-fibre nociceptor are likely to be sensitive to irritant chemicals.

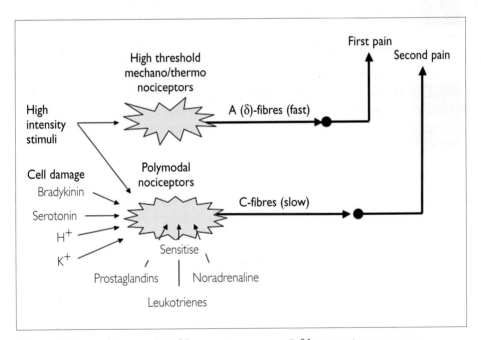

Figure 1.11: A-fibre and C-fibre nociceptors. C-fibre nociceptors are directly activated by certain substances released by cell damage and are also sensitised by certain chemical by-products of cell damage. Receptor subtypes exist for A-fibre and C-fibre nociceptors, and it is likely that there is some overlap in stimuli for activation between groups

- *C-fibre nociceptors:* these are particularly sensitive to chemicals released during actual cell damage such as hydrogen ions (H^+), potassium ions (K^+), serotonin (5-HT) and bradykinin. They also respond to noxious thermal and mechanical events. C-fibre nociceptor activity contributes to 'second' or 'slow' pain sensations that help to guard the injury from further damage (e.g. 'dull' and 'aching' pain sensations, *Figure 1.10*). Significant proportions of C-fibre nociceptors are polymodal and can respond to thermal, mechanical, and chemical stimuli. It is now emerging that many A-fibre nociceptors are also polymodal (Drew and Wood, 2004; Koltzenburg, 2004; Meyer *et al*, 2006).

It should be remembered that these subdivisions are gross oversimplifications. Furthermore, high intensity noxious stimuli will also activate non-nociceptive mechano and thermo receptors which have low thresholds of activation. Activity in these non-nociceptive mechano and thermo receptors will also 'flavour' the sensation of pain experienced by a person. In fact, when the nociceptive system becomes sensitised, these non-nociceptive receptors begin to signal noxious events.

Transmission

Afferent neurons transmit nerve impulses from nociceptors to the spinal cord and/or brainstem (peripheral transmission), and from the spinal cord and/or brainstem to higher centres in the brain (central transmission) (*Figure 1.10*) (Craig and Dostrovsky, 1999; Raja *et al*, 1999; Willis, 2004; Dostrovsky and Craig, 2006).

- *Peripheral transmission:* A-fibre nociceptors transmit impulses in small diameter myelinated A-delta afferents with conduction velocities above $2\,ms^{-1}$, usually in the $25\,ms^{-1}$ range. Impulses in these 'fast' transmitting nociceptive fibres reach the brain 'first' and contribute to the sharp, severe, localised pain immediately following a noxious event ('fast' or 'first' pain). C-fibre nociceptors transmit impulses in small diameter unmyelinated C afferents with conduction velocities below $2\,ms^{-1}$, usually in the $0.5\,ms^{-1}$ range. Impulses in these 'slow' transmitting nociceptive fibres reach the brain after the A-fibre impulses and contribute to the dull aching, less severe, spreading pain (i.e. 'slow' or 'second' pain). Most peripheral nociceptive afferents terminate in the superficial part of the dorsal horn and synapse directly or indirectly (via interneurons) on to central nociceptive transmission cells.

Peripheral nociceptive afferents release a variety of excitatory substances, although all tend to use glutamate as their main neurotransmitter.

- **Central transmission:** central nociceptive transmission neurons transmit information about noxious stimuli from the spinal cord and brainstem to higher brain centres such as the thalamus (spinothalamic tracts [STT]), the brainstem reticular formation (spinoreticular tract [SRT]), and the hypothalamus and forebrain (spinohypothalamic tract [SHT]). Activity in central nociceptive transmission neurons is increased with input from nociceptive peripheral afferents and excitatory interneurons. Activity in central nociceptive transmission neurons is reduced (modulated), with input from low threshold (innocuous) mechano and thermal afferents (segmental modulation), and/ or descending pain inhibitory pathways arising from the brain (extrasegmental modulation). Interneuron-releasing inhibitory neurotransmitters, such as gamma-amino-butyric-acid (GABA), glycine and metenkephalin are often involved (see 'The suppressed pain state', _pp. 31–32_). Under certain circumstances activity in central nociceptive transmission neurons is enhanced (amplified) by peripheral and/or central mechanisms (see 'The sensitised pain state', _pp. 21–22_).

There are a variety of central nociceptive transmission neurons (Dostrovsky and Craig, 2006). Often they are generalised as nociceptive specific neurons (NS) and wide dynamic range neurons (WDR, _Figure 1.13_; Price, 2007). NS neurons respond to high intensity stimuli and are predominantly found in lamina I of the dorsal horn. They send information in the spinothalamic tract which provides a rapid and direct route to sensory areas of the cerebrum (e.g. somatosensory cortex). This provides information regarding the intensity, quality, and location of the noxious stimuli. WDR neurons respond to non-noxious and noxious stimuli arriving in A-fibre and C-fibre nociceptors and A-fibre 'touch' afferents. This is why they are called 'wide dynamic range' neurons. WDR neurons are predominantly found in lamina V of the dorsal horn and form multi-synaptic pathways projecting to the reticular formation in the brainstem and to the limbic system and the frontal lobes in the cerebrum. Central nociceptive transmission neurons also project to the hypothalamus via spinohypothalamic tracts to elicit sympathetic changes, as described earlier (Price, 2007).

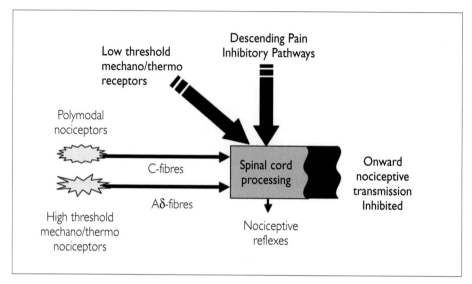

Figure 1.12: Endogenous pain suppression systems. Activity in low threshold mechanoreceptors (i.e. touch and rubbing), and thermoreceptors (i.e. cooling or warming), and descending pain inhibitory pathways will inhibit ongoing activity in central nociceptive transmission cells

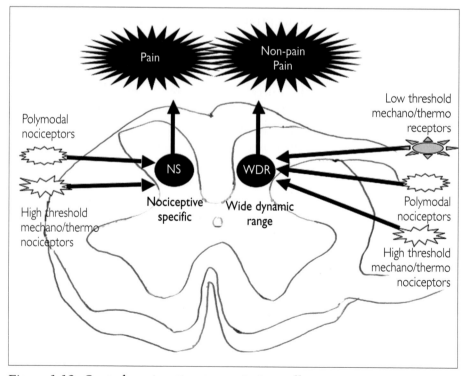

Figure 1.13: Central nociceptive transmission cells

Perception

Perception is the process by which we become aware of something through our senses. The primary somatosensory cortex of the cerebrum (SI) contributes to pain sensation by processing incoming information to aid discrimination of the location and nature of noxious and non-noxious stimuli impinging on the body. SI receives an ordered neural input of body parts from the opposite side of the body (*Figure 1.14*). Body parts with high densities of sensory receptor cells have proportionately larger areas of SI devoted to processing incoming information and are better at discriminating two discrete stimuli (i.e. are more sensitive) (Penfield, 1968; Flanders, 2005).

Removal of nociceptive transmission neurons or removal of the

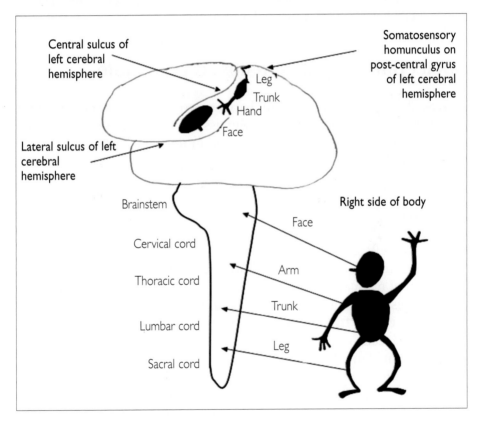

Figure 1.14: Somatotopic ('body map') representation in the central nervous system. Somatosensory pathways project in an ordered manner to areas of the contralateral somatosensory cortex (SI). Large areas of the cortex process input from body parts that have fine discrimination, creating a distorted body map termed a homunculus

somatosensory cortex itself does not improve pain in the long term, suggesting that pain perception is more complex than simply activating a single pain centre in the brain. Neuroimaging techniques, such as positron emission tomography (PET) and functional magnetic resonance imaging (fMRI) have revealed activity in a variety of brain areas when healthy humans experience experimentally-induced pain. Interestingly, different patterns of brain activity are seen in patients with persistent pain suggesting that there is no brain 'centre' devoted to pain experience, and that different areas become active in different situations. Areas commonly seen to be involved in pain processing are the thalamus and somatosensory cortex (sensory dimensions), the cingulate gyrus and insula (affective dimensions), and the prefrontal cortex (cognitive dimensions) (Gybels and Tasker, 1999; Ingvar and Hsieh, 1999; Davis, 2000; Treede *et al*, 2000; Bushnell and Apkarian, 2006).

Nociception — the sensitised pain state

Increased sensitivity to stimuli happens to cutaneous, visceral and muscle tissue and helps to protect the tissue from further damage. This sensitisation occurs in the periphery and in the central nervous system (*Figure 1.15*).

Peripheral sensitisation

Damage to cells causes the accumulation of algesic (pain producing) substances in the extracellular fluid which reduces the threshold of activation of nociceptors at the site of injury (peripheral sensitisation). These algesic substances have leaked out of damaged cells; have been synthesised from precursors that have themselves leaked out of damaged cells; or have arrived in the area as a result of plasma extravasation ('outside vessel') or lymphocyte migration.

In addition, nerve impulses generated by nociceptor activity invade the distal branches of the nociceptor free nerve endings, causing the release of substance P and other trophic chemicals into the surrounding tissue (*Figure 1.16*). Some of these chemicals may play a critical role in wound healing. This 'chemical soup' produces vasodilatation, increased blood flow, increased permeability of blood vessels, and plasma extravasation associated with inflamed tissue (i.e. redness, heat, and swelling). Some algesic substances such

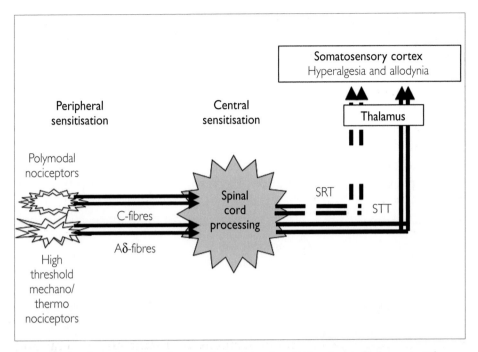

Figure 1.15: Peripheral and central sensitisation following cell damage. The thresholds of activation of peripheral and central nociceptive cells are lowered as a result of sensitisation causing an amplification of provoking stimuli

as Bradykinin, 5-HT, H^+, and K^+ activate nociceptors leading to pain in the absence of external stimuli. Other substances, such as prostaglandins, leukotrienes, noradrenaline, adenosine, adenosine 5-triphosphate (ATP), and nitric oxide, sensitise nociceptors by lowering their threshold of activation (Levine and Reichling, 1999; Meyer *et al*, 2006).

A basic knowledge of this neurobiology of peripheral sensitisation helps to understand how some pain-relieving drugs work. Non-steroidal anti-inflammatory drugs (NSAIDs, e.g. ibuprofen and diclofenac) and aspirin, reduce the production of prostaglandins by inhibiting cyclo-oxygenase (Cox), an enzyme that speeds up the formation of prostaglandins (PG) from arachidonic acid. Cox exists as two isozymes (Cox-I and Cox-II), and drugs that selectively inhibit Cox-II were developed to reduce side-effects and improve efficacy. These Cox-II inhibitors (e.g. celecoxib, etodolac, rofecoxib and meloxicam) are used for short-term treatment of acute inflammation in joints caused by arthritis, but there has been concern about risks to the cardiovascular system. The effect of NSAIDs on bleeding and inflammation needs to be carefully evaluated prior to use for mild wound pain (Seibert *et al*, 1994; McQuay and Moore, 2006).

Central sensitisation

Damage to cells resulting in persistent C-fibre nociceptor activity also reduces the threshold of activation of central nociceptive transmission cells (central sensitisation) through the process of 'wind-up' (Dickenson *et al*, 2004; Herrero, 2007). Wind-up is a form

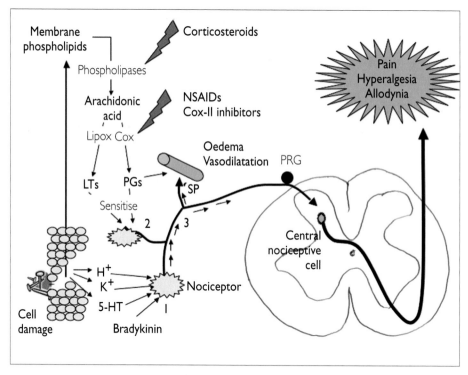

Figure 1.16: Peripheral events following tissue damage. Substances resulting from tissue damage can directly activate nociceptors [1] or can cause the synthesis of leukotrienes [LTs] and prostaglandins [PGs] that act to sensitise nociceptors [2]. Impulses also invade the nerve endings of the nociceptor and release substance P [SP]. This inflammatory soup causes vasodilatation and plasma extravasation [3]. Enzymes that catalyse the synthesis of LT and PG (i.e. phospholipases, lipoxases [Lipox] and cyclo-oxygenases [Cox]) can be inhibited by corticosteroids, NSAIDs and Cox-II inhibitors. PRG = posterior root ganglion

of temporal summation whereby central nociceptive transmission neurons increase in their response to repeated C-fibre nociceptor activity, as would occur in post-burn or post-abrasion injuries. Wind-up contributes to hyperalgesia by making central nociceptive transmission neurons hyperexcitable and they may even begin to respond to non-noxious stimuli to produce allodynia (*Figure 1.17*). This is what makes wound dressing changes so unpleasant. Central nociceptive transmission neurons also expand their receptive fields so that they begin to respond to stimuli applied to sites on the body that do not normally activate the neuron producing secondary hyperalgesia. It is believed that secondary hyperalgesia in the healthy tissue that surrounds the injury is due to central sensitisation, rather than local accumulation of algesic substances at the site of damage (Cousins and Power, 1999; Doubell *et al*, 1999; Raja *et al*, 1999; Treede, 2007).

The pharmacology of central sensitisation is complex and involves many neurochemicals. Two common neurotransmitters released by peripheral nociceptive afferents on to central nociceptive transmission cells are glutamate, which is an excitatory amino acid

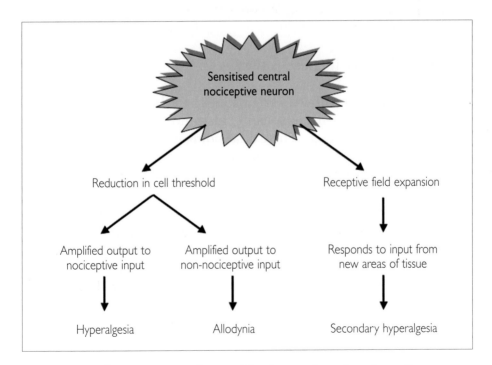

Figure 1.17: Characteristics of a sensitised central nociceptive cell

and substance P, which is an excitatory peptide. These substances sensitise the central nociceptive transmission cell by binding to and activating a variety of membrane receptors such as NMDA (N-methyl D-aspartate) receptors (e.g. glutamate), and neurokinin receptors (e.g. substance P). Many other transmitter substances are also involved in central sensitisation such as calcitonin-gene-related-peptide (CGRP), somatostatin, vasoactive intestinal polypeptide (VIP), nerve growth factor, and nitric oxide (Yaksh, 1999).

The NMDA receptor may have a crucial role in the transition between acute and chronic pain (Dickenson and Sullivan, 1987). Activation of the NMDA receptor by sustained release of glutamate and substance P from peripheral nociceptive afferent terminals results in an influx of Ca^{++} into the central nociceptive transmission neuron (*Figure 1.18*). This changes the neuron's excitability and structure, and results in reorganisation of neuronal circuitry within the central nervous system (central neuroplasticity). Ketamine is a drug that acts as an NMDA antagonist and has been used to try to prevent central sensitisation occurring in pains due to severe burns. Furthermore, pre-emptive analgesics have also been used prior to surgical procedures to reduce potential long-term consequences of central sensitisation associated with post-operative pain.

Descending pain facilitatory pathways

It is now known that pathways originating in the brainstem can increase responses of neurons in the spinal cord to noxious and non-noxious stimuli (Suzuki *et al*, 2005). These descending pain facilitatory pathways enhance the magnitude of pain sensation by reducing the threshold of activation of NS and WDR neurons. Descending pain facilitatory pathways improve the detection and localization of potentially dangerous stimuli and contribute to sensitized pain states which helps to protect the injury. However, persistent activity in descending pain facilitatory pathways may lead to persistent hypersensitivity that serves no useful purpose (Pertovaara 2007, Zhuo 2007).

Pain resulting from treatments, such as wound dressing and debridement, are clear examples of allodynia and hyperalgesia and result from peripheral and central sensitisation. The importance of effectively managing pain during these procedures cannot be over emphasised, because failure to do so may result in persistent central sensitisation, which may be irreversible.

The persistent (chronic) pain state

A sensitised nociceptive system should return to its pre-sensitised state once tissue has healed and pain should disappear. However, many patients experience persistent pain. This may occur before the formation of a wound, in non-healing wounds, or after a wound has healed. Persistent pain may be nociceptive (i.e. via activation of nociceptors), neuropathic (i.e. when there has been nerve damage), or both.

Persistent nociceptive pain

Nociceptive wound pain is more common than neuropathic wound pain and, as described previously, results from ongoing activation and sensitisation of nociceptors. Persistent nociceptive pain may be due to an underlying condition causing ongoing ischaemia, oedema, or tissue damage, as seen with arterial and venous disease. Alternatively, it may result from the prolonged time for healing of a serious trauma such as a post-burn injury, whereby peripheral and central sensitisation will persist and the wound will be sensitive to provoking stimuli. Nociceptive wound pain is receptive to primary analgesic agents such as paracetamol, NSAIDs, local anaesthetics, and opioids. Failure to manage the pain may cause long-term changes in the structural and functional organisation of the nociceptive system, so that pain persists even if the wound eventually heals.

In situations where there has been nerve damage, pain may persist despite the apparent healing of tissue, as seen with post-amputation pain or post-herpetic neuralgia. In these circumstances, pain may result from pathophysiology of the nociceptive system.

Neuropathic pain

Pain resulting from nerve damage is called neuropathic pain. Nerve lesions may affect sensory, motor and autonomic fibre and, as a consequence, response to treatment can be variable. Factors contributing to neuropathic pain include:

- hypersensitive central nociceptive cells
- abnormal inputs to central nociceptive cells
- reflex muscle spasm

- ectopic impulse generation
- loss of large diameter afferent (segmental) inhibition.

There may also be sympathetic hyperactivity (Devor and Seltzer, 1999; Hansson *et al*, 2001). However, persistent central sensitisation seems to be a common factor following injury to neural tissue.

In general, neuropathic pain is characterised by unusual sensations such as numbness, paraesthesia, and pains that are described as shooting, burning, electrical, and deep aching. Mechanical and/or

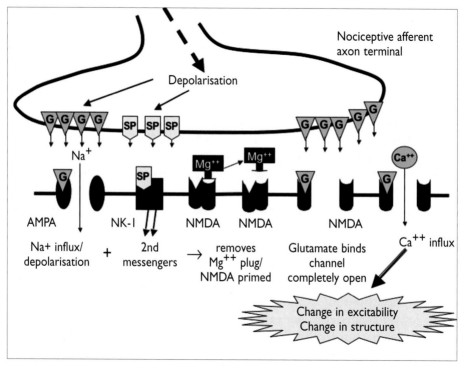

Figure 1.18: Activation of NMDA receptors. Depolarisation of the nociceptor afferent terminal causes the release of glutamate [G] and substance P [SP], either from separate fibres or co-released by the same fibre. Glutamate activates AMPA receptors and depolarises the central nociceptive neuron, whereas substance P activates neurokinin receptors [NK-1] activating second messengers. Simultaneous activation of AMPA and NK-1 receptors removes an Mg^{++} plug from the NMDA receptor and, if glutamate activates the NMDA receptor, Ca^{++} channels will open. An influx of Ca^{++} to the post synaptic central nociceptive cell leads to long-term changes in the structural and functional abilities of the central nociceptive cell

thermal allodynia and hyperalgesia may be present. Neuropathic wound pain is difficult to control and antidepressant or anti-epileptic drugs are commonly used.

Lesions of peripheral nerves, as seen in diabetes or in deep wounds, are termed peripheral neuropathies. If nerves are severed distal to the cell body, a clump of regenerating neuronal sprouts termed a neuroma may form. The neuroma, and the posterior root ganglion, may be spontaneously active (i.e. ectopic firing) producing pain in the absence of stimuli (*Figure 1.19*). Neuromas are also sensitive to provoking stimuli and may generate excessive amounts of nerve impulses which further sensitise central nociceptive transmission neurons. This may explain why some wounds that appear to have healed, may still be painful to touch, as seen in post-amputation stump pain (Wall and Gutnick, 1974; Dickenson *et al*, 2001).

When nerves are damaged proximal to the cell body, central nociceptive transmission neurons may become spontaneously active because of the lack of normal afferent input (*Figure 1.20*). This may explain why an injury that appears to have healed may still generate background pain, as seen following brachial plexus avulsions when a person's arm is paralysed and insensitive to touch, yet manifests a severe aching pain. Phantom limb pains are also likely to result in part from spontaneously active central nociceptive transmission neurons (Devor and Seltzer, 1999).

Reorganisation of central neuronal circuits
One consequence of nerve damage is structural and functional re-organisation of the nervous system. For example, areas of SI with input from intact nerves invade areas of SI that have lost their input due to nerve damage. This may explain some of the unusual phantom sensations experienced post amputation, such as stroking the cheek with a Q-tip generating a phantom hand sensation. This is because the area of SI receiving input from the cheek invades the neighbouring area of SI which has lost its normal input from the amputated hand (Flor *et al*, 1995; Flor *et al*, 1998; Montoya *et al*, 1998). Nerve damage can also lead to a predominance of activity in descending pain facilitatory pathways causing persistent hypersensitivity (Pertovaara, 2007; Zhuo, 2007).

Neuropathy with diminished sensation
Sometimes tissue does not heal, yet there is no pain because nerve damage has caused diminished sensation, as seen with neuropathic

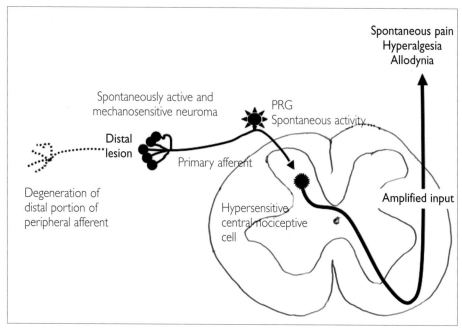

Figure 1.19: Nerve lesions distal to the posterior root ganglion. Distal lesions cause ectopic impulse generation at neuroma and the posterior root ganglion [PRG] leading to central sensitisation

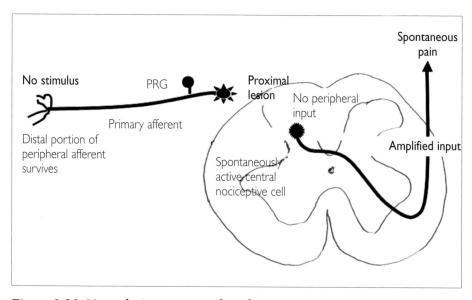

Figure 1.20: Nerve lesions proximal to the posterior root ganglion (PRG). Ectopic impulse generation arises in central nociceptive cells due to the lack of peripheral input

foot ulcers (neuropathy with diminished sensation). Peripheral neuropathy, as seen with diabetes, can result in sensory loss causing ulceration at sites of high pressure. Neuropathies of motor and autonomic nerves may cause abnormal plantar pressure and anhydrotic skin which is prone to fissuring, resulting in neuropathic foot ulcers. Interestingly, neuropathic foot ulcers are often painless despite the potential for peripheral and central sensitisation (Edmonds and Foster, 2006).

The suppressed pain state — pain modulation

Pain sensation can be reduced by suppressing activity in the nociceptive system, as described by the Gate Control Theory of Pain (Melzack and Wall, 1965). The 'pain gate' is a metaphor to explain regulation of nociceptive information. The 'pain gate' can be opened by activity in peripheral nociceptor transmission pathways (A-fibre and C-fibre nociceptors), leading to onward transmission of noxious information to the brain. When the 'pain gate' is closed, onward transmission of noxious information from the spinal cord to the brain is suppressed. This can be achieved in two ways (*Figure 1.21*).

Activity in non-noxious afferents (segmental modulation)

Activity in peripheral non-noxious afferents (e.g. touch and pressure) can be generated by rubbing healthy skin close to painful or damaged areas of the body, hence the term 'rubbing pain better'. Passing low intensity electrical currents across the skin can also be used to activate non-noxious afferents in a technique called transcutaneous electrical nerve stimulation (TENS). In many respects, TENS 'electrically rubs pain away'. It has been shown that TENS reduces central nociceptive transmission neurons by activating inhibitory interneurons in the spinal cord that release GABA and enkephalins (Garrison and Foreman, 1994; Sluka and Walsh, 2003; Johnson, 2008).

Activity in descending pain inhibitory nerve pathways (extrasegmental modulation)

Activity in neural pathways arising from areas in the brainstem, such as the periaqueductal grey (PAG) and the raphe nuclei, causes inhibition of central nociceptive transmission neurons through pre- and post-synaptic inhibitory mechanisms (*Figure 1.21*). These descending pain inhibitory nerve pathways involve many transmitter substances including opioid peptides (predominantly acting on μ receptors, but also on δ and κ receptors), serotonin, and noradrenaline (acting on α−2 receptors). These receptors are prime targets for many analgesic drugs such as opioids (e.g. morphine) and amitryptiline (Fields and Basbaum, 1999; Dubner and Ren, 2004; Villanueva and Fields, 2004).

Deep structures and referred pain

Nociceptors in deep structures

Most knowledge about pain physiology comes from studies on superficial structures like the skin. However, wounds may penetrate deeper somatic structures, such as skeletal muscle, connective tissue of the joints and bone. Wounds may also penetrate visceral structures, such as cardiac muscle and smooth muscle of the gastrointestinal, renal and vascular systems. Nociceptors in the skin evolved to signal encounters with external stimuli and tend to generate discrete localised pains, promoting escape behaviour. Nociceptors in deep tissue have evolved to detect noxious stimuli resulting from stretching and imbalances in fluid pH, and they tend to generate pain that is dull and less well localised, as characterised in *Table 1.3*.

The principles of nociception are similar for deep structures as they are for the skin. A-fibre and C-fibre nociceptors become sensitised in the presence of tissue damage and contribute to spontaneous pain, allodynia and hyperalgesia. However, nociceptors in deeper structures vary considerably in the type of stimuli that provoke activity. Skeletal muscle is sensitive to contraction in the presence of ischaemia, which can generate a deep aching pain, as seen with limb ischaemia and associated ischaemic ulcers. These pains can have both nociceptive and neuropathic elements. Visceral structures are sensitive to twisting, distension and chemical irritants (e.g. stomach acid), but are relatively insensitive to cutting, heat or pinching (Cousins, 1987; Blendis, 1999; Procacci *et al*, 1999; Mense and Simons, 2001; Schaible, 2006; Bielefeldt and Gebhardt, 2006).

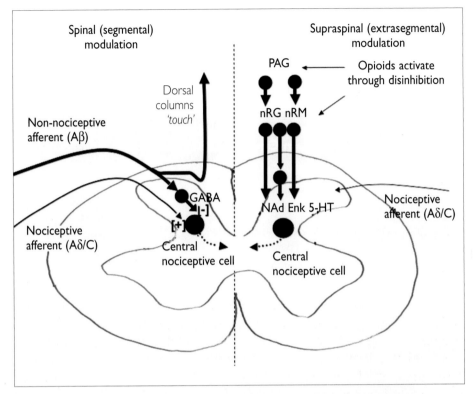

Figure 1.21: Endogenous pain suppression systems. Ongoing activity in central nociceptive transmission cells can be reduced by inhibitory interneurons [-] releasing GABA and possibly met-enkephalin [Enk] at a segmental level, or by activity in the periaqueductal gray [PAG], nucleus raphe magnus [nRM] and nucleus raphe gigantocellularis [nRG] at an extrasegmental level releasing noradrenalin [NAd], 5-hydroxytryptamine [5-HT] and enkephalin [Enk]. Excitatory = [+]; Inhibitory = [-]

Physiology of referred pain

The poor localisation of deep somatic and visceral pain is due to fewer central nociceptive transmission neurons dedicated to visceral input. Damage in deep structures may result in referred pain which is felt at sites remote from tissue damage and pathology. Pathology in deep structures often produces characteristic patterns of skin sensitivity and pain because their afferents are bundled in nerves that primarily innervate structures like the skin. Often pain is referred to the cutaneous area innervated by the same spinal segment (dermatome) as the visceral structure, because visceral and cutaneous afferents supply the same central nociceptive transmission neuron (*Figure 1.22*). The brain interprets the afferent input as arising from cutaneous structures because of the higher proportion of cutaneous afferents converging on central nociceptive transmission neurons. Referred pain can confuse the clinician and the patient (Fields, 1987; Borowczyk, 2007).

Table 1.3: The characteristics of pain arising from superficial versus deep tissue (adapted from **Cousins**, 1987)		
	Superficial	Deep
Tissues	Cutaneous, mucous	Cardiac, skeletal and smooth muscle. Fascia, periosteum, joint and connective tissue
Intensity of pain	Often related to severity of damage	Diminished relationship to severity of damage
Quality of pain	Sharp, pricking, stinging	Dull, sore, aching
Location of pain	Precise and localised Strong relationship with stimulus/injury	Diffuse and poorly localised Weaker relationship with stimulus/injury and may be referred to another area of the body
Temporal aspects of pain	Often constant rather than periodic	Often periodic and may build to peak intensity
Related symptoms	Autonomic symptoms occur if damage is moderate and involves deep tissue	Autonomic symptoms often present — nausea, vomiting, sweating, palpitations

Summary

Wound pain is a major issue for patients and may be associated with underlying pathology and/or treatment, such as debridement or dressing changes. Under-treatment of wound pain is a problem and leads to a state of physiological stress which is detrimental to health. Nowadays, the concept of pain being generated by a 'hard wired pain pathway' is outdated, as many biopsychosocial factors influence the way that we experience pain. The neural circuitry that detects stimuli that produce actual or potential tissue damage is called the nociceptive system. In its normal (control) state, the nociceptive system detects noxious stimuli and generates protective reflex responses and pain so that we can avoid the noxious stimuli in the future. In its suppressed state, the nociceptive system reduces pain to enable us to escape from threatening situations even if there is appreciable tissue damage. In its sensitised state, the nociceptive system amplifies pain and this

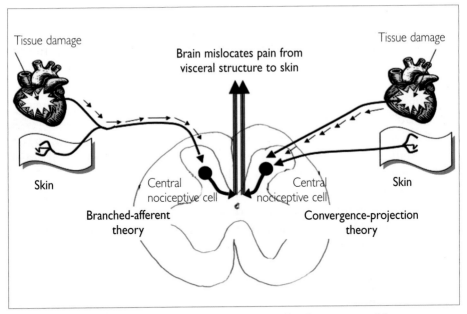

Figure 1.22: The physiology of referred pain. The brain is unable to discriminate the source of the incoming noxious information [arrows] as arising from visceral structures (e.g. heart) or somatic structures (e.g. skin). This tends to result in pain referred to the somatic structures

aids tissue healing by discouraging behaviours that may cause further tissue damage. Some pain-relieving treatments try to block nociceptive information reaching the brain by interfering with the nociceptive system. NSAIDs and local anaesthetics are good examples. Some pain-relieving treatments interact with our own endogenous pain-relieving systems. Opioids and TENS are good examples. Persistent wound pain may be nociceptive in origin, resulting from ongoing activation of nociceptors and sensitisation of the nociceptive system. This may be due to an underlying condition or a prolonged time for a wound to heal. Persistent wound pain may be neuropathic in origin, resulting from damage to nerves. It will cause irreversible functional and structural reorganisation in the nervous system.

References

Baron R, Janig W (2004) The role of the sympathetic nervous system in pain processing. In: Villanueva L, Dickenson AH, Ollat H, eds. *The Pain System in Normal and Pathological States: A Primer for Clinicians'*

Progress. Pain Research and Management, Volume 31. IASP Press, Seattle: 193–210

Basbaum A (2004) Molecular approaches to understanding the anatomical substrates of nociceptive processing. In: Villanueva L, Dickenson AH, Ollat H, eds. *The Pain System in Normal and Pathological States: A Primer for Clinicians' Progress. Pain Research and Management, Volume 31.* IASP Press, Seattle: 123–137

Bielefeldt K, Gebhart GF (2006) Visceral pain: basic mechanisms In: McMahon SB, Koltzenburg M, eds. *Wall and Melzack's Textbook of Pain.* Elsevier Churchill Livingstone, Edinburgh: 721–36

Blendis LM (1999) Abdominal pain. In: Wall PD, Melzack R, eds. *Textbook of Pain.* Churchill Livingstone, Edinburgh: 603–19

Borowczyk J (2007) Visceral Referred Pain In: Schmidt RF, Willis WD, eds. *Encyclopedia of Pain.* Springer, Berlin: 2645–7

Bushnell MC, Apkarian AV (2006) Representation of pain in the brain. In: McMahon SB, Koltzenburg M, eds. *Wall and Melzack's Textbook of Pain.* Elsevier Churchill Livingstone, Edinburgh: 107–24

Cousins M (1987) Visceral disease. In: Andersson S, Bond M, Mehta M, Swerdlow M, eds. *Chronic Non-cancer Pain.* MTP Press Limited, Lancaster: 119–30

Cousins M, Power I (1999) Acute and post-operative pain. In: Wall PD, Melzack R, eds. *Textbook of Pain.* Churchill Livingstone, Edinburgh: 447–92

Craig AD (2006) Emotions and psychobiology. In: McMahon SB, Koltzenburg M, eds. *Wall and Melzack's Textbook of Pain.* Elsevier Churchill Livingstone, Edinburgh:231–39

Craig AD, Dostrovsky JO (1999) Medulla to thalamus. In: Wall PD, Melzack R, eds. *Textbook of Pain.* Churchill Livingstone, Edinburgh: 183–214

Davis KD (2000) Studies of pain using functional magnetic resonance imaging. In: Casey KL, Bushnell MC, eds. *Pain Imaging. Pain Research and Management, Volume 18.* IASP Press, Seattle: 195–210

Devor M, Seltzer Z (1999) Pathophysiology of damaged nerves in relation to chronic pain. In: Wall PD, Melzack R, eds. *Textbook of Pain.* Churchill Livingstone, Edinburgh: 129–64

Dickenson AH, Sullivan AF (1987) Evidence for a role of the NMDA receptor in the frequency dependent potentiation of deep rat dorsal horn nociceptive neurones following C fibre stimulation. *Neuropharmacol* 26: 1235–8

Dickenson AH, Matthews EA, Suzuki R (2001) Central nervous system mechanisms of pain in peripheral neuropathy. In: Hansson PT, Fields

HL, Hill RG, Marchettini P, eds. *Neuropathic Pain: Pathophysiology and Treatment. Pain Research and Management, Volume 21.* IASP Press, Seattle: 85–106

Dickenson AH, Suzuki R, Matthews EA, Rahman W, Urch C, Seagrove L, Rygh L (2004) Balancing excitations and inhibitions in the spinal circuits. In: Villanueva L, Dickenson AH, Ollat H, eds. *The Pain System in Normal and Pathological States: A Primer for Clinicians' Progress. Pain Research and Management Volume 31.* IASP Press, Seattle: 79–105

Dostrovsky JO, Craig AD (2006) Ascending projection systems. In: McMahon SB, Koltzenburg M, eds. *Wall and Melzack's Textbook of Pain.* Elsevier Churchill Livingstone, Edinburgh: 187–203

Doubell TP, Mannion RJ, Woolf CJ (1999) The dorsal horn: state-dependent sensory process, plasticity and the generation of pain. In: Wall PD, Melzack R, eds. *Textbook of Pain.* Churchill Livingstone, Edinburgh: 165–82

Drew LJ, Wood JN (2004) Molecular mechanisms of noxious mechanosensation. In: Villanueva L, Dickenson AH, Ollat H, eds. *The Pain System in Normal and Pathological States: A Primer for Clinicians' Progress. Pain Research and Management, Volume 31.* IASP Press, Seattle: 3–27

Dubner R, Ren K (2004) Brainstem modulation of pain after inflammation. In: Villanueva L, Dickenson AH, Ollat H, eds. *The Pain System in Normal and Pathological States: A Primer for Clinicians' Progress. Pain Research and Management, Volume 31.* IASP Press, Seattle: 107–22

Edmonds ME, Foster AVM (2006) Diabetic foot ulcers. *Br Med J* **332**: 407–10

European Wound Management Association (EWMA) (2002) Position Document: *Pain at wound dressing changes.* London: MEP Ltd

Fields HL (1987) Pain from deep tissues and referred pain. In: Fields HL, ed. *Pain.* McGraw-Hill Book Company, New York: 79–97

Fields HL, Basbaum AI (1999) Central nervous system mechanisms of pain modulation. In: Wall PD, Melzack R, eds. *Textbook of Pain.* Churchill Livingstone, Edinburgh: 309–30

Flanders M (2005) Functional somatotopy in sensorimotor cortex. *Neuroreport* **16**(4): 313–6

Flor, H, Elbert T, Knecht S (1995) Phantom-limb pain as a perceptual correlate of cortical reorganization following arm amputation. *Nature* **375**: 482–4

Flor H, Elbert T, Muhlnickel W (1998) Cortical reorganization and phantom phenomena in congenital and traumatic upper-extremity amputees. *Exp Brain Res* **119**: 205–12

Freedman G, Entero H, Brem H (2004) Practical treatment of pain in patients with chronic wounds: pathogenesis-guided management. *Am J Surg* **188**: 31S–35S

Garrison DW, Foreman RD (1994) Decreased activity of spontaneous and noxiously evoked dorsal horn cells during transcutaneous electrical nerve stimulation (TENS). *Pain* 58: 309–15

Gybels JM, Tasker RR (1999) Central neurosurgery. In: Wall PD, Melzack R, eds. *Textbook of Pain*. Churchill Livingstone, Edinburgh: 1307–39

Hansson PT, Lacerenza M, Marchettini (2001) Aspects of clinical and experimental pain: The clinical perspective. In: Hansson PT, Fields HL, Hill RG, Marchettini P, eds. *Neuropathic Pain: Pathophysiology and treatment. Pain Research and Management, Volume 21.* IASP Press, Seattle: 1–18

Herrero JF (2007) Wind-Up of Spinal Cord Neurons. In: Schmidt RF, Willis WD, eds. *Encyclopedia of Pain*. Springer, Berlin: 2668–70

Ingvar M, Hsieh JC (1999) The image of pain. In: Wall PD, Melzack R, eds. *Textbook of Pain*. Churchill Livingstone, Edinburgh: 215–33

Johnson MI (2008) Transcutaneous electrical nerve stimulation. In: Watson T, ed. *Electrotherapy: Evidence-based practice*. Churchill Livingstone, Edinburgh: 22–96

Levine JD, Reichling DB (1999) Peripheral mechanisms of inflammatory pain. In: Wall PD, Melzack R, eds. *Textbook of Pain*. Churchill Livingstone, Edinburgh: 59–84

Koltzenburg M (2004) Thermal sensitivity of sensory neurons. In: Villanueva L, Dickenson AH, Ollat H, eds. *The Pain System in Normal and Pathological States: A Primer for Clinicians' Progress. Pain Research and Management, Volume 31.* IASP Press, Seattle: 29–43

Krasner D (1995) The chronic wound experience. *Ostomy/Wound Management* 41: 20–5

McCaffery M (1983) *Nursing the Patient in Pain*. Harper & Row, London

McQuay HJ, Moore A (2006) NSAIDS and Coxibs: clinical use. In: McMahon SB, Koltzenburg M, eds. *Wall and Melzack's Textbook of Pain*. Elsevier Churchill Livingstone, Edinburgh: 471–80

Melzack R (1975) The McGill Pain Questionnaire: major properties and scoring methods. *Pain* 1: 277–99

Melzack R, Katz J (1999) Pain measurements in persons in pain. In: Wall PD, Melzack R, eds. *Textbook of Pain*. Churchill Livingstone, Edinburgh: 409–26

Melzack R, Wall P (1965) Pain mechanisms: A new theory. *Science* 150: 971–9

Melzack R, Wall PD (1988) *The Challenge of Pain*. Penguin Books, London

Mense S, Simons D (2001) *Muscle Pain. Understanding its nature, diagnosis, and treatment*. Lippincott Williams and Wilkins, Philadelphia

Merskey H, Bogduk N (1994) *Classification of Chronic Pain: Descriptions of Chronic Pain Syndromes and Definitions of Pain Terms.* 2nd edn. IASP Press, Seattle

Meyer RA, Ringkamp M, Campbell JN, Raja SN (2006) Peripheral mechanisms of cutaneous nociception. In: McMahon SB, Koltzenburg M, eds. *Wall and Melzack's Textbook of Pain.* Elsevier Churchill Livingstone, Edinburgh: 3–34

Moffat CJ, Franks PJ, Hollingworth H (2002) Understanding wound pain and trauma: an international perspective. In: *European Wound Management Association Position Document. Pain at wound dressing changes.* Medical Education Partnership Limited, London: 2–7

Montoya P, Ritter K, Huse E, Larbig W, Braun C, Topfner S *et al* (1998) The cortical somatotopic map and phantom phenomena in subjects with congenital limb atrophy and traumatic amputees with phantom limb pain. *Eur J Neurosci* **10**: 1095–102

Penfield W (1968) Engrams in the human brain. Mechanisms of memory. *Proc R Soc Med* **61**: 831–40

Pertovaara A (2007) Descending modulation and persistent pain In: Schmidt RF, Willis WD, eds. *Encyclopedia of Pain.* Springer, Berlin: 564–7

Price DD (2007) Spinothalamic tract neurons, in deep dorsal horn. In: Schmidt RF, Willis WD, eds. *Encyclopedia of Pain.* Springer, Berlin: 2278–82

Price P, Fagervik-Morton H, Mudge EJ, *et al* (2008) Dressing-related pain in patients with chronic wounds: an international patient perspective. *Int Wound J* **2**: 159–71

Procacci P, Zoppi M, Maresca M (1999) Heart, vascular and haemopathic pain. In: Wall PD, Melzack R, eds. *Textbook of Pain.* Churchill Livingstone, Edinburgh: 621–40

Raja SN, Meyer RA, Ringkamp M *et al* (1999) Peripheral neural mechanisms of nociception. In: Wall PD, Melzack R, eds. *Textbook of Pain.* Churchill Livingstone, Edinburgh: 11–58

Ready L, Edwards WT (1992) *Management of Acute Pain: A practical guide.* IASP Press, Seattle

Schaible H-G (2006) Basic mechanisms of deep somatic tissues In: McMahon SB, Koltzenburg M, eds. *Wall and Melzack's Textbook of Pain.* Elsevier Churchill Livingstone, Edinburgh: 621–34

Scheinfeld N (2005) The law on the failure to treat pain. *Ostomy Wound Management* **51**(11A suppl): 7–8

Seibert K, Zhang Y, Leahy K *et al* (1994) Pharmacological and biochemical demonstration of the role of cyclooxygenase 2 in inflammation and pain. *Proc Natl Acad Sci USA* **91**: 12013–7

Sluka KA, Walsh D (2003) Transcutaneous electrical nerve stimulation: basic science mechanisms and clinical effectiveness. *J Pain* 4(3): 109–21

Suzuki R, Rygh LJ, Dickenson AH (2005) Bad news from the brain: descending 5-HT pathways that control spinal pain processing. *Trends Pharmacol Sci* 25(12): 613–7

Treede RD (2007) Allodynia (Clinical, Experimental). In: Schmidt RF, Willis WD, eds. *Encyclopedia of Pain*. Springer, Berlin: 49–52

Treede RD, Apkarian AV, Bromm B (2000) Cortical representation of pain: functional characterization of nociceptive areas near the lateral sulcus. *Pain* 87: 113–19

Villanueva L, Fields HL (2004) Endogenous central mechanisms of pain modulation. In: Villanueva L, Dickenson AH, Ollat H, eds. *The Pain System in Normal and Pathological States: A Primer for Clinicians' Progress. Pain Research and Management, Volume 31*. IASP Press, Seattle: 223–46

Willis WD (2004) Spinothalamocortical Processing of Pain. In: Villanueva L, Dickenson AH, Ollat H, eds. *The Pain System in Normal and Pathological States: A Primer for Clinicians Progress. Pain Research and Management, Volume 31*. IASP Press, Seattle: 155–78

Wall PD, Gutnick M (1974) Properties of afferent nerve impulses originating from a neuroma. *Nature* 248: 740–3

Woolf CJ (1987) Physiological, inflammatory and neuropathic pain. *Adv Tech Stand Neurosurg* 15: 39-62

Woolf CJ (2007) Central sensitization: uncovering the relation between pain and plasticity. *Anesthesiology* 106(4): 864–7

Woolf CJ (1994) The dorsal horn: state-dependent sensory processing and the generation of pain. In: Wall PD, Melzack R, eds. *Textbook of Pain*. Churchill Livingstone, Edinburgh: 101–12

Woolf CJ, Salter MW (2000) Neuronal plasticity: increasing the gain in pain. *Science* 288: 1765–9

Yaksh T (1999) Central pharmacology of nociceptive transmission. In: Wall PD, Melzack R, eds. *Textbook of Pain*. Churchill Livingstone, Edinburgh: 253–308

Zhuo M (2007) Descending facilitatory systems. In: Schmidt RF, Willis WD, eds. *Encyclopedia of Pain*. Springer, Berlin: 559–63

CHAPTER 2

DRESSING-RELATED PAIN IN PATIENTS WITH CHRONIC WOUNDS: AN INTERNATIONAL PATIENT PERSPECTIVE

Patricia Price, Hilde Fagervik-Morton, Elizabeth Mudge, Hilde Beele, José Contreras-Ruiz, Theis Huldt Nystrøm, Christina Lindholm, Sylvie Meaume, Britta Melby-Østergaard, Yolanda Peter, Marco Romanelli, Salla Seppänen, Thomas Serena, Gary Sibbald, Jose Verdú Soriano, Wendy White, Uwe Wollina, Kevin Woo, Carolyn Wyndham-White, Keith Harding

This cross-sectional international survey assessed patients' perceptions of their wound pain. A total of 2018 patients (57% female) from 15 different countries with a mean age of 68.6 years (SD = 1/4 15.4) participated. The wounds were categorised into ten different types with a mean wound duration of 19.6 months (SD = 51 8). For 2018 patients, 3361 dressings/compression systems were being used, with antimicrobials being reported most frequently ($n = 605$). Frequency of wound-related pain was reported as 32.2%, 'never' or 'rarely', 31.1%, 'quite often' and 36.6%, 'most' or 'all of the time', with venous and arterial ulcers associated with more frequent pain ($P = 0.002$). All patients reported that 'the wound itself' was the most painful location ($n = 1840$). When asked if they experienced dressing-related pain, 286 (14.7%) replied 'most of the time' and 334 (17.2%) reported pain 'all of the time'; venous, mixed and arterial ulcers were associated with more frequent pain at dressing change ($P < 0.001$). Eight hundred and twelve (40.2%) patients reported that it took < 1 hour for the pain to subside after a dressing change, for 449 (22.2%) it took 1–2 hours, for 192 (9.5%) it took 3–5 hours and for 154 (7.6%) patients it took more than 5 hours. Pain intensity was measured using a visual analogue scale (VAS) (0–100) giving a mean score of 44.5 (SD = 30.5, $n = 1981$). Of the 1141 who reported that they generally took pain relief, 21% indicated that they did not feel it was effective. Patients were asked to rate six symptoms associated with living with a chronic wound; 'pain' was given the highest mean score of 3.1 ($n = 1898$). In terms of different types of daily activities, 'overdoing things' was associated with the highest mean score (mean = 2.6, $n = 1916$). During the stages of the dressing change procedure; 'touching/handling the wound' was given the highest mean score of 2.9, followed by cleansing and dressing removal (n = 1944). One thousand four hundred and eighty-five (75%) patients responded that they liked to be actively involved in their dressing changes, 1141 (58.15%) responded that they were concerned about the long-term side-effects of medication, 790 (40.3%) of patients indicated that the pain at dressing change was the worst part of living with a wound. This study adds substantially to our knowledge of how patients experience wound pain and gives us the opportunity to explore cultural differences in more detail.

Introduction

In recent years there has been growing evidence that the experience of living with a chronic wound has a huge impact on a patient's quality of life (Franks *et al*, 1994; Price and Harding, 1996). One of the consistent findings, particularly in the qualitative work that has been completed, is that pain is one of the symptoms that patients find particularly distressing (Charles, 1995; Ebbeskog and Ekman, 2001; Rich and McLachlan, 2003).

Pain is a universal experience and there is little debate that pain is undeniably subjective and individual (Brennan *et al*, 2007). Very early pain research emphasised the mechanical nature of pain, such as the withdrawal of the relevant body part from the noxious stimulus as a result of nerve activation (Horn and Munafo, 1998). However, the Gate Control Theory (Melzack and Wall, 1982) finally acknowledged the role of brain processes in the perception of pain that helped to explain how injured athletes can continue to compete without noticing pain, while raised anxiety can result in the experience of pain without any apparent injury. The integration of the physiological and psychological aspects of pain in a single model mirrors the broader change in clinical practice away from a purely medical approach towards holistic patient care.

Healthcare professionals are now starting to recognise the importance of addressing the issue of wound pain, as evidenced by the European Wound Management Association Position Document (EWMA, 2002) on pain, the dedication of a supplement of *Ostomy Wound Management* to this topic (Reddy *et al*, 2003) and the Consensus Document on minimising pain at wound dressing-related procedures launched at the World Union of Wound Healing Societies meeting (WUWHS, 2004). However, evidence exists across many health states that there is a major gap between an increasingly sophisticated understanding of the pathophysiology of pain and widespread inadequate pain management (Brennan *et al*, 2007).

Although only limited work has been completed on pain in chronic wounds, much of this has focused on pain at dressing change. In a multinational survey, practitioners consistently rated dressing removal as the time of greatest pain (Moffatt *et al*, 2002). It is understandable why this should be the initial point of interest; we all have memories of gauze-based dressings sticking to childhood injuries and the distraction techniques our parents used to stop us from crying. Given that patients with leg ulcers are usually elderly with particularly fragile skin, the removal of dressings that stick to the wound may well be the most painful part of the dressing procedure (Briggs and Torra i Bou, 2002). Adding to this the potential impact of dressings on trauma to the surrounding skin, the drive to produce a dressing that is almost painless to remove with little or no impact on the surrounding tissue is to be applauded. One of the ways in which manufacturers are attempting to limit the potential for pain on dressing removal is by the use of alternative adhesives for atraumatic dressings.

Although work has been completed on the views of healthcare professionals and their perception of patient pain experiences, little research has been completed to gain the views of patients directly. Differences in personal, familial and cultural backgrounds can lead to great variation in the experience and expression of pain by individuals (Koral and Craig, 2001). The potential for making errors during the pain assessment procedure is vast, particularly if we are not aware of the cultural norms within which our patients or we are operating.

This is the report of the second phase of a two-phase study on the understanding of patients' experiences of pain related to living with chronic wounds. Phase I was a qualitative phase conducted in three countries that formed the basis of the questionnaire to be used in Phase II: the data from this phase has been presented (Mudge, 2007).

This part of the study aimed to:

- explore the extent of problems related to pain and dressing-related procedures

- compare pain experiences between wound types (wounds of the lower leg and foot) across a range of countries.

Methods

A patient survey was conducted in 15 countries (Australia, Belgium, Canada, Denmark, Finland, France, Germany, Italy, Mexico, Norway, Spain, Sweden, Switzerland, UK and the US). Participants were asked to complete a questionnaire, developed following a qualitative phase of the study (Mudge, 2007). This was a cross-sectional, descriptive questionnaire design, providing predominantly quantitative data. The draft questionnaire was piloted on ten patients with chronic wounds, but only minor amendments were needed. The questionnaire was translated through expert linguists in each of the relevant countries, with substantial experience of medical-related translation: all regional questionnaires were back-translated into English to confirm accuracy.

Sample

Each country identified a national coordinator who agreed to take part in the survey, who asked nurses or physicians from their respective professional wound care societies to participate. The aim was to encourage nurses or physicians from a range of locations to participate in order to get a sample that was reflective of the geographical and socioeconomic factors relevant to each country: a total target sample of 2000 was sought. It was anticipated that a substantial number of healthcare professionals in each country would agree to participate and each nurse/physician was asked to invite up to ten patients from their caseload to participate.

Patients over the age of 18 years with an active, chronic wound, who were able and willing to participate and who had experienced discomfort/pain related to their chronic wound within the previous month were eligible for participation. Wherever possible, the patients were asked to complete the questionnaires independently; however, the relevant nurse/physician/healthcare volunteer could assist with the process by reading the questions if necessary: however, all participating nurses or physicians were asked not to complete the questionnaire to reflect their own views of the patients' experiences. The inclusion criteria were deliberately broad to ensure that the full range of patients with these wound types could participate.

Procedure

All nurses or physicians who agreed to participate in the study were asked to ensure that the appropriate permissions were in place for their facility. Nurses or physicians were given written instructions related to the procedure; a country specific telephone number and email address was provided in order to answer specific questions that arose.

Nurses or physicians were encouraged to explain the procedure to the patient and leave the questionnaire for the patient to complete in their own time, collecting the questionnaire at the same visit. In exceptional circumstances, when this process was difficult, the patient could be provided with a stamped addressed envelope to return the questionnaire (although this option was not used during the data collection). If the patient required help with completing the questionnaire, the nurse or physician was asked to complete this task with the patient after the clinical part of the visit was completed. Each member of staff was asked to ensure that the questionnaire had been fully completed and that the free text was readable. The national coordinator agreed the details of the process for their own country and ensured that the text was translated into English before returning the forms for analysis. All data were collected between March and October 2007.

Ethical issues

All necessary permissions were sought for this phase of the study from the relevant ethical review committees in each country. Participation was entirely voluntary and patient care was not affected in any way by their decision to participate or to choose not to participate. Patients were not mentioned specifically by name or referred to in any way, and any papers based on the study will only include summary data related to the way in which responses reflect the comments made by participants. Data were kept in locked filing cabinets and accessed only by those directly involved with the analysis of data and the lead investigators in each country. Original data will be kept for six months after the final publications are prepared and then destroyed.

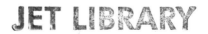

Data analysis

Data were entered into a database (SPSS Inc., Chicago, IL, USA version 14) for quantitative analysis. Four researchers were involved in the input of data, following appropriate training. In instances where data were missing, these were coded as 999 while not applicable was coded as 888. In any case where the respondent placed a tick between two values these were always rounded down, thus underestimating the scores; this did not account for more than ten items in any one variable. Data quality checks were carried out to ensure consistency in data input and coding; these included visual checks, random checks for complete patient input, systematic checks for invalid entries and values outside the expected range. Any inconsistencies were resolved by checking back with the original questionnaire. The data were summarised by wound type and by country using frequency counts and appropriate summary statistics. All comparative analysis was performed on a descriptive or conservative basis, as this was not a hypothesis testing study. Where appropriate, chi-square was used for categorical data, the median test for data where one variable was nominal and the other ordinal and Friedman test for within patient analyses for ordinal data with multiple groups; parametric, continuous variables were analysed using one-way analysis of variance. Alpha was set at 0.05. Open comments were translated, transcribed and analysed using content analysis by two independent researchers to ensure a high level of reliability in coding the data. Several categories had to be coded to reduce the number of options provided in the raw data: data coding schedules were devised through multidisciplinary expert groups, with confirmation by the two researchers involved in coding the data.

Results

Results were obtained for 2018 patients in the specified time, from 15 different countries: 57% of participants were female (*Table 2.1*). For a survey of this size, missing data are to be expected, but this varied across the variables. Nineteen patients did not give their gender (0 9%), while 61 (3%) did not identify a wound type. The return rate of questionnaires varied by country over the 15 countries involved in the project, with the biggest contribution from Italy (19.5%) and the smallest from an individual country being Belgium (1.3%). The average age of participants was 68.6 years (min = 19, max = 101, SD = 15.4) across all countries (35 sets of missing data, 1.7%). Given the size of the data set, these results will focus on the results over all countries by wound type.

There was a range of wound aetiologies from the 15 participating countries; 46.3% were leg ulcers of known aetiology with a further 19.8% recorded as ulcers of unknown aetiology (66% in total). Around 20% of the sample was diabetic foot ulcers or pressure ulcers, with a further 7% made up of surgical, trauma wounds or burns and the final 7% classified as 'other', which included a range of conditions, such as *pyoderma gangrenosum*.

Table 2.1: Gender distribution by country			
Country	Male	Female	Total (%)
Australia	40	41	81 (4.1)
Belgium	11	15	26 (1.3)
Canada	56	44	100 (5.0)
Denmark	60	61	121 (6.1)
Finland	27	37	64 (3.4)
France	45	95	140 (7.0)
Germany	69	78	147 (7.4)
Italy	165	225	390 (19.5)
Mexico	85	74	159 (8.0)
Norway	40	61	101 (5.1)
Spain	63	89	152 (7.6)
Sweden	36	63	99 (5.0)
Switzerland	48	59	107 (5.4)
UK	73	123	196 (9.8)
USA	48	68	116 (5.8)
Total	866	1133	1999* (100)

*There were 19 sets of missing data.

Table 2.2 outlines the frequency of patients presenting with their first wound experience. Across all wound types, 43.8% of patients were describing their first experience of a wound. Thirty-three questionnaires reported this was unknown, with a further 6.6% of questionnaires where these data were missing.

The average wound duration across all wound types was 19.6 months (SD = 51.8 months), with a large range from >1 month to 65 years. There was also a large range within each wound type, as outlined in *Table 2.3*, with the burn wounds having the longest mean duration of 43.9 months.

A vast range of dressings was used across wound types and across countries; these have been categorised into ten generic dressing types and are presented in *Table 2.4*. Some patients had as many as seven different dressings and compression systems reported as being used at the time the questionnaire was completed.

Antimicrobials were reported as used most frequently (*n* = 650) and were the leading dressing type used in Australia, Belgium, Canada, Finland, Germany, Italy, Spain, UK and USA. These country-specific trends and international preference for use of specific products

Table 2.2: First experience of ulceration by wound type			
First ulcer for patient	Not first ulcer	Unknown	Total
Venous	204	350	7	561
Arterial	84	103	4	191
Mixed	47	83	1	131
Diabetic	75	117	2	194
Pressure	98	69	9	176
Ulcer (unknown)	174	189	7	370
Surgical	35	15	1	51
Trauma	44	23	1	68
Burns	10	4	0	14
Other	52	76	1	129
Total	823 (43·8)	1029 (54·6)	33 (1·8)	1885* (100)

*There were 133 cases of missing data.

highlight the popularity of antimicrobial dressings in some countries and potential reimbursement issues and availability. Furthermore, antimicrobial dressings were also the overall largest group of dressing type reported by respondents as causing 'more pain' (14%; silver dressings – n = 52 and iodine-based dressings – n = 39), whereas the most common dressings listed as causing 'less pain' were a soft silicone polyurethane foam, a hydrofibre and a foam with topical ibuprofen. It is, however, important to interpret these findings with caution at this stage as further analyses about dressing choice needs to be conducted.

The experience of pain

Patients were asked 'Do you have any pain related to your ulcer?', with five response options ranging from 'never' to 'all the time' (*Table 2.5*). Only 7% of patients reported that they never felt wound pain regardless of wound type: 30 of the 136 patients in that category, had

Table 2.3: Duration of wound by wound type (in months)			
Wound type	N	Mean	SD
Venous	553	22.9	45.1
Arterial	189	16.8	33.7
Mixed	131	28.2	44.7
Diabetic	191	12.1	21.8
Pressure	174	11.9	22.1
Ulcer (unknown)	366	22.7	72.2
Surgical	52	7.5	7.5
Trauma	71	26.7	129.9
Burns	13	43.9	97.2
Other	130	15.3	27.2
Missing	37	8.8	18.7
Total	1907*	19.6	51.79

*There were 111 cases of missing data.

Table 2.4: Total generic dressings used

Ulcer	Classification of dressing												Total
	AF	NAF	C	AM	A	HCD	F	O	AD	NAD	None	M	
Venous	110	42	161	184	89	43	2	287	3	82	16	12	1031
Arterial	31	24	16	70	45	20	0	104	1	17	1	4	333
Mixed	31	11	17	46	30	10	0	83	—	20	1	2	252
Diabetic	31	20	14	78	32	10	1	89	4	43	9	4	335
Pressure	44	29	9	39	44	20	1	71	—	25	2	3	288
Unknown aetiology	69	33	59	134	64	13	8	214	4	47	2	11	658
Surgical	12	3	4	16	12	4	1	22	0	7	0	0	81
Trauma	9	11	8	19	11	9	0	35	0	12	1	0	115
Burns	1	1	2	5	2	2	0	9	0	0	—	0	23
Other	25	12	16	59	28	13	1	69	0	20	0	2	245
Total	363	186	306	650	357	144	14	983	14	273	33	38	3361

AF, adhesive foam; NAF, non-adhesive foam; C, compression; AM, antimicrobial; A, alginate; HCD, hydrocolloid; F, film; O, other; AD, adhesive dressing; NAD, non-adhesive dressing; None, no dressing currently being used; M, missing data.

ulcers of unknown origin. At the other end of the scale, 16.1% of patients reported that they had wound pain all the time; 119 (38%) of these were recorded as having venous ulcers and 16.9% as having ulcers of unknown origin. If the response options are collapsed into three categories then across all wound types, 32.2% reported pain as 'never' or 'rarely', 31.1% reported pain 'quite often' and 36.6% reported pain 'most' or 'all of the time'. There are statistical differences between the wound types, with venous, arterial and mixed ulcers reporting more frequent pain experiences.

When asked 'where is the pain when it is most painful?', 1840 patients replied (the 178 sets of missing data included the 140 who replied that they did not experience any pain, so this question did not apply to them). Although patients were asked to limit their answers to three options, some patients gave additional details such as 'surrounding skin and elsewhere' (*Table 2.6*). The largest group of patients across all wound types indicated that the wound itself was the most painful and this pattern was consistent for each wound type.

Table 2.5: Experience of pain by wound type					
Wound type	Never	Rarely	Quite often	Most of the time	All of the time
Venous	23	127	177	125	119
Arterial	10	44	64	48	31
Mixed	6	37	39	32	18
Diabetic	26	55	62	35	23
Pressure	18	52	53	28	30
Ulcer (unknown)	30	107	116	80	53
Surgical	11	11	20	2	8
Trauma	2	21	25	12	10
Burns	0	3	8	4	0
Other	10	33	41	32	21
Total (%)	136 (7)	490 (25.2)	605 (31.2)	398 (20.5)	313 (16.1)

Median x² = 26·42; P = 0·002.

Table 2.6: Location of pain by wound type

Wound type	In the wound	Wound and surrounding skin	Surrounding skin	Surrounding skin and elsewhere	Radiating elsewhere
Venous	291	8	159	1	95
Arterial	100	3	54	1	27
Mixed	82	0	22	1	22
Diabetic	99	3	37	1	45
Pressure	94	1	39	0	26
Ulcer (unknown)	168	6	102	0	90
Surgical	30	1	11	1	5
Trauma	37	2	13	0	14
Burns	8	0	4	0	3
Other	77	0	29	1	22
Total (%)	986 (53.59)	24 (1.3)	470 (25.54)	6 (0.33)	349 (18.97)

Patients were asked how frequently, if ever, they experienced pain at dressing change. The biggest category response was 'rarely' at 28.5% (*Table 2.7*). If the categories are collapsed into three responses, then 45.3% experience pain at dressing change 'never' or rarely', 21.9% have pain at dressing change 'quite often' and 31.9% report pain at dressing change 'most to all' of the time.

In terms of overall results, there is a statistically significant difference between the groups when analysed using the median test, with venous, mixed and arterial ulcers being associated with more frequent experiences of pain at dressing change.

Patients were asked to report how long it took any pain that they experienced at dressing change to subside, using a four-point scale of time, but also giving a 'not applicable' option for those who reported that they never felt pain at dressing change. Although there are 100 sets of missing data for this question, 1918 responded with only 311 of those reporting that the question was 'not applicable'. Overall, 812 (40.2%) respondents reported that it took less than one hour for the pain to subside, for 449 (22.2%) it took 1–2 hours, for 192 (9.5%)

it took three to five hours, and for 154 (7.6%) patients it took more than five hours. One thousand eight hundred and sixty-three of these patients also identified their wound type (*Table 2.8*).

When the results are analysed using the median test, there is a statistically significant difference between the wound types, with patients with mixed ulcers taking the longest time for the pain to resolve.

Words that describe the pain experience

Patients were asked to complete a variation of the McGill Short-form Pain Questionnaire, which was translated and back-translated across the relevant languages used in the countries involved. These terms can be summarised into two main domains, known as 'sensory' and 'affective'. The scores for each word in the tool by wound type for each country are presented in the appendices. *Table 2.9* presents the summaries for the two domains for all 1999 patients who provided data for this part of the questionnaire (sensory scale from 0 to 30, affective scale from 0 to 12: on both scales a higher score indicated more severe

Table 2.7: Pain at dressing change by wound type					
Wound type	Never	Rarely	Quite often	Most of the time	All of the time
Venous	75	150	144	96	109
Arterial	23	59	40	35	40
Mixed	14	32	33	25	28
Diabetic	55	56	46	20	22
Pressure	40	55	32	20	33
Ulcer (unknown)	68	125	77	54	61
Surgical	16	16	12	5	4
Trauma	10	27	21	5	7
Burns	2	4	5	2	2
Other	23	30	33	24	28
Total (%)	326 (16.78)	554 (28.51)	443 (21.95)	286 (14.72)	334 (17.19)

levels of pain), overall and by wound type. For both domains there are statistically significant differences between the wound types; there are more patients above the median with venous, arterial, mixed ulcers and burns than in the other groups in the sensory domain; and more patients above the median for venous, mixed and other ulcers in the affective domain. These data confirm the quantitative data collected in other items, whereby patients with venous ulceration rated their pain more extremely.

Pain intensity

Patients were asked to identify the intensity of pain they had experienced in the previous week, leading up to the time of completing the questionnaire, on a VAS scale of 0–100 (where 0 meant no pain, 100 signified worst possible pain). The full range of the scale was used, with a mean score of 44.5 over all patients and a standard deviation of

Table 2.8: Time for the pain to resolve after dressing change by wound type (n = 1863)

Wound type	Less than 1 hour	1–2 hours	3–5 hours	More than 5 hours	Not applicable
Venous	231	149	65	47	69
Arterial	76	44	24	15	29
Mixed	39	36	19	19	17
Diabetic	93	35	12	12	35
Pressure	83	34	3	17	37
Ulcer (unknown)	155	82	38	25	64
Surgical	23	9	2	2	12
Trauma	28	11	8	3	14
Burns	8	3	1	0	3
Other	55	31	14	10	22
Total (%)	791 (42.46)	434 (23.3)	186 (9.98)	150 (8.05)	302 (16.21)

Median $x^2 = 31.61$; $P = 0.001$.

Table 2.9: Sensory and affective domain scores by wound type

	N	Mean	Median	Range
Sensory	1999	8.78	7	0–30
Venous	571	9.84	8	0–30
Arterial	196	9.43	7	0–30
Mixed	131	9.41	8	0–30
Diabetic	199	8.38	7	0–30
Pressure	181	7.5	4	0–30
Ulcer (unknown)	384	8.19	6	0–30
Surgical	54	5.88	4	0–24
Trauma	71	6.76	5	0–23
Burns	15	7.73	8	1–19
Other	137	8.92	6	0–27
Affective	1999	2.43	0	0–12
Venous	571	2.78	1	0–12
Arterial	196	2.54	0·5	0–12
Mixed	131	3.20	1	0–12
Diabetic	199	2.01	0	0–12
Pressure	181	2.06	0	0–12
Ulcer (unknown)	384	2.16	0	0–12
Surgical	54	1·37	0	0–12
Trauma	71	1.53	0	0–11
Burns	15	1.86	0	0–9
Other	137	2.78	1	0–12
Total (%)	1999			

Median test x^2(sensory) $= 39·13, P<0·001$ (affective) $= 30·31, P<0·001$

30.5 ($n = 1981$). *Figure 2.1* suggests that the full range of the scale was used by the majority of patients within each of the different wound types, with the lowest median for surgical wounds and the highest for mixed ulcers and burn wounds. These data provide further support to the McGill data, suggesting that patients with leg ulcers and burns experience the greatest pain intensity.

Pain relief

Patients were also asked if they took any pain relief for their wound-related pain. Although 12 participants did not provide an answer to this question (0.6%), 1303 (64.6%) of the total sample stated they did take pain relief. Seven patients reported that this question did not apply to them, whereas five reported that the pain relief worked 'sometimes'. Of the 1671 patients who replied, 1141 (68%) stated that when they did take pain relief it generally made a difference, while 530 (32%)

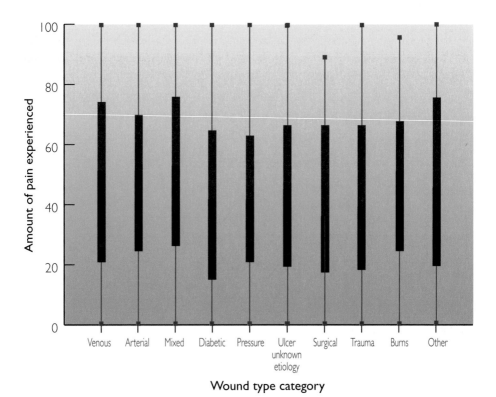

Figure 2.1: Box plot for visual analogue socres by wound type. Median is represented by the bold line within the box. $F_{9,911} = 2.36$, $P = 0.012$

recorded that pain relief did not generally work (this is the variable with the largest amount of missing data at 17.3%). If the results for the two questions on pain relief are put together, then of the 1670 who replied to both questions the results are slightly different (*Table 2.10*): 83% of those who were taking pain relief for their wound pain stated

Table 2.10: Taking pain relief and associated effectiveness

	Does medication relieve wound pain? (%)		
	Yes	No	Total (%)
Pain relief taken?			
Yes	1058 (83)	217 (17)	1275 (100)
No	82 (21)	313 (79)	395 (100)
	1140	530	1670

$x^2 = 538.9$, $d.f. = 1$, $P < 0.001$

Table 2.11: Taking pain relief by wound type

	Pain relief taken		
Wound type	Yes (%)	No (%)	Total (%)
Venous	376 (65.6)	197 (34.4)	573
Arterial	140 (71.1)	57 (28.9)	197
Mixed	90 (68.7)	41 (31.3)	131
Diabetic	117 (58.5)	83 (41.5)	200
Pressure	98 (53.8)	84 (42.6)	182
Ulcer (unknown)	269 (69.9)	116 (30.1)	385
Surgical	29 (53.7)	25 (46.3)	54
Trauma	43 (60.6)	28 (39.4)	71
Burns	11 (73.3)	4 (26.7)	15
Other	97 (70.3)	41 (29.7)	138
Total (%)	1270 (65.3)	676 (34.7)	1946 (100.0)

that it worked, but 79% of those who were not taking pain relief (at the time they completed the questionnaire) felt it was not effective (which could explain why they were not taking any medication at the time).

Pain relief medication was also analysed by wound type (*Table 2.11*). The wound types associated with the highest levels of taking pain relief are burns, arterial and other wounds. The highest levels of not taking medication are associated with surgical wounds and pressure ulcers.

Symptom experience

Patients were asked to rate six symptoms on a five-point scale (1, not a problem, 5, a major problem); the frequencies overall participants can be seen in *Table 2.12*. 'Difficulties in not being able to take a bath or a shower' was recorded with the highest number of responses, indicating that this was a major problem, with 'pain' as the second most frequently cited major problem.

If, however, the symptoms are ordered by their mean scores (based on the results of 1898 participants who responded to all of the items), then 'pain' is given the highest mean score of 3.08. The order of the symptoms in terms of being problematic (over all respondents) is pain, impaired mobility, difficulties in bathing, leakage, odour and slippage of the dressing or bandage.

Participants were also asked to rate the levels of pain associated with different types of daily activities, again using a five-point scale (1, no pain; 5, very painful). In terms of the frequency of 'very painful', then the highest frequency was recorded for pain due to wound infection (*Table 2.13*). If, however, the symptoms are ordered by their mean scores (based on the results of 1916 participants who responded to all of the items), then 'overdoing things' is associated with the highest mean score. The order of activities in terms of associated pain is overdoing things, sleeping at night, pain at dressing change, pain associated with infection and pain on waking.

Participants were asked to rate the different stages of the dressing change procedure, again using a 1–5 scale (1, no pain; 5, very painful). The part of the dressing change procedure with the highest frequency of 'very painful' was 'touching/handling the wound' followed by 'cleansing' (*Table 2.14*). If, however, the symptoms are ordered by their mean scores (based on the results of 1944 participants who responded to all of the items), then 'touching/handling the wound' is given the highest mean score of 2.97. The order of the symptoms in terms of pain during dressing change is touching/handling the wound, cleansing, dressing removal, time after application of new dressing and time waiting for dressing change.

Participants were asked whether there were products available that make the dressing change procedure less painful. Six hundred and twenty patients (of the 1785 who responded to this question) indicated that products could make a difference. When asked for specific examples of such products, a huge range of products were highlighted; items identified by at least ten patients can be found in *Table 2.15*.

Of the 1360 patients who responded to the question 'If there was one thing that you would like healthcare professionals to do for you to help with your pain at/during dressing-related procedures, what would it be?', 61 patients (4.5%) reported that they were satisfied with the treatment provided regardless of whether they experienced pain and 22 patients (1.6%) stated that they did not experience any pain at/during dressing-related procedures. The majority of participants (495 patients; 36.4% of those who answered) answered that they felt the healthcare professionals in charge of their care could do nothing to help with their pain at/during dressing-related procedures; similarly, 144 patients (10.6%) did not know of anything that would be beneficial to their care. For those who provided suggestions for healthcare professionals, 14.9% of patients felt that analgesics/ anaesthetics would be beneficial, 8.0% emphasised a wish for the healthcare professional to be careful and gentle during treatment, 4.0% of patients highlighted the importance of being consulted with, listened to, communicated with and distracted from the dressing-related procedures, to have their dressing soaked/moistened before removal (3.3%) and not to rush the procedures (2.3%). Advice on avoiding touching and/or scrubbing the wound, ensuring consistency and sound quality of care and a wish to have the wound washed with water were also reported (2.1%, 1.5% and 0.9% respectively).

Attitudes to living with pain

Patients were asked to describe the extent to which they agreed with four statements on dressing change pain and living with long-term use of pain medication, using a five-point Likert Scale (strongly agree to strongly disagree) (*Table 2.16*). One thousand four hundred and

Table 2.12: Experience of different wound symptoms

	1 (not a problem)	2	3	4	5 (a major problem)	Total (responses to this item)	Mean (n=1898)	Median	Range
Odour	1209	285	191	132	153	1970	1.85	1	1–5
Leakage	716	393	359	238	281	1987	2.49	2	1–5
Pain	430	344	359	329	516	1978	3.08	3	1–5
Impaired mobility	566	293	335	349	430	1973	2.89	3	1–5
Bathing	686	235	282	260	521	1984	2.86	3	1–5
Bandage slippage	1188	312	212	143	120	1975	1.84	1	1–5

Table 2.13: Experience of pain by daily activity

	1 (no pain)	2	3	4	5 (very painful)	Total (responses to this item)	Mean (n=1916)	Median	Range
Waking up	949	348	280	206	206	1989	2.19	2	1–5
Overdoing things	657	348	333	332	300	1970	2.63	2	1–5
Sleeping (night)	730	343	355	276	282	1986	2.52	2	1–5
Dressing changes	699	420	341	248	277	1985	2.5	2	1–5
Pain due to wound infection	843	268	237	282	330	1960	2.49	2	1–5

Table 2.14: Experience of pain with different parts of the dressing change procedure

	1 (no pain)	2	3	4	5 (very painful)	Total	Mean (n = 1944)	Median	Range
Waiting for dressing change	1193	337	233	123	93	1979	1.78	1	1–5
Dressing/tape removal	867	417	299	212	189	1984	2.23	2	1–5
Cleansing	592	413	351	297	326	1979	2.68	2	1–5
Touching/handling the wound	440	430	327	333	456	1986	2.97	3	1–5
Re-application of new dressing	974	431	265	181	132	1983	2.03	2	1–5
Time after new dressing applied	827	454	335	228	139	1983	2.20	2	1–5

Table 2.15: Generic products/techniques that make the dressing change procedure less painful

Generic products/techniques	Number of participants who suggested product/technique	Generic products/techniques	Number of participants who suggested product/technique
Creams or gels	44	Hydrocolloids	13
Non-adhesive dressings	39	Hydrogels	13
Local anaesthesia	34	Topical application of anaesthetic cream or gel	11
Moisten dressings before removing them	20	Foam dressings	10
Moist dressings	17	Morphine or other pain-relieving medication	10
Gauze	13		

Table 2.16: Attitudes to living with wound pain						
	Strongly agree	Agree	Uncertain	Disagree	Strongly disagree	Total
I like to be actively involved in the process of changing my dressings	716	769	197	178	125	1985
I am concerned about long-term use of pain medication (e.g. side-effects)	463	678	320	307	194	1962
Overall, the pain experienced while having the dressing change is the worst part of living with an ulcer	318	472	295	607	270	1962
Overall, wound pain at other times is the worst part of living with an ulcer	567	687	278	288	143	1963

seventy-five (75%) of patients responded that they liked to be actively involved in their dressing changes, 1141 (58.15%) responded that they were concerned about the long-term side-effects of medication, 790 (40.3%) of patients indicated that the pain at dressing change was the worst part of living with a wound (with a relatively even split across the categories); however, 1254 (63.8%) agreed that pain at other times was the worst pain of living with an ulcer.

Discussion

This is one of the biggest international surveys of the patient perspective of chronic wound pain, particularly focusing on dressing-related procedures. The results suggest that wound type is a strong indicator of wound pain experiences, across all cultural groups, with venous and arterial ulcers associated with more frequent pain. It is unfortunate that so many responses only identified the aetiology of the wound as 'ulcer', as this group had to be analysed separately, which may have underestimated the pain experience of this group; the missing information may reflect insufficient documentation, or that a large number of patients do not have a complete diagnosis. Direct comparison between groups is also confounded by the inclusion of unexpected wound types (e.g. burns and trauma): given the inclusion criteria for the study, we can only conclude that these are wounds that have become 'chronic' because of the duration of the wound, rather than original cause. The findings also suggest that most wound pain is experienced in the wound itself, with >30% of all wound types experiencing dressing-related pain most or all of the time; approximately 60% of the sample reported that it took longer than one hour for this pain to resolve.

Participants were asked to rate the different components of the dressing change procedure: the category with the highest mean score was 'touching/handling', followed by cleansing and dressing removal. These data support the growing awareness of pain associated with the cleansing part of the procedure (Lindholm, 2007; Woo *et al*, 2007). The response option 'touching/handling' was included as it was frequently brought up during the qualitative section of this study; however, interpretation of this option has associated difficulties. The response options for this question were waiting for dressing change; dressing/tape removal; cleansing; touching/handling the wound; reapplication of new dressing; time after the new dressing is applied. Many of these options follow a time-course related to the dressing change procedure; however, touching/handling the wound may have involved several stages of the process and not just the time when the wound is uncovered. This is particularly important to recognise given the translation issues, which may have resulted in a possible misunderstanding.

Although every effort was made to ensure that the translation process was rigorous, the importance of language in the assessment of pain cannot be underestimated. Languages often have a completely different vocabulary for descriptions of noxious substances; languages also differ in the number of words used to describe pain, as well as the emotional content of the pain descriptors (Koral and Craig, 2001). Some difficulties were experienced in translating the component parts of the McGill Short-Form questionnaire, particularly into Spanish. However, the study focused predominantly on developed countries influenced by European health perspectives (Europe, Australia and North Americas). The variation in sample size from different countries is partly explained by the time taken to gain all appropriate permissions, with those countries that were able to gain approval earlier recruiting the most patients. Future studies may consider a limit on participation by country to avoid any particular cultural view being overrepresented. If the study were to be conducted in a broader range of countries, the questionnaire would need to be reconsidered in the light of dominant cultural beliefs regarding the medical system and treatment of illness.

Participants were asked to rate their pain experience compared with other symptoms that can be experienced when living with a chronic wound: in this instance, pain was considered the biggest problem. However, in direct comparison with other activities of daily life, 'generally overdoing' was considered the most painful event. This shows that questions related to pain may need to be set in context to ensure appropriate comparisons are made. The responses to the use of analgesia reflect studies in other health states, such that many of the participants responded that they were concerned about the long-term side-effects of taking analgesia (58%). However, 64% reported that they took pain relief for the wound pain, with 82% suggesting that the medication they took was effective, which is considerably higher than previous studies (Quirino *et al*, 2003).

Conclusion

This present survey has documented that chronic wound pain, particularly as part of dressing-related procedures, is common with variations in pain experience related to wound aetiology and 64% of patients taking analgesia to cope with their pain experiences. However, further analysis is necessary to fully understand the role of cultural diversity on pain assessment and management. Research has already shown that views about health that are dominant in Western cultures do not prevail in other parts of the world (Tu, 1980); the same applies to the meanings attached to the experience of pain and how we perceive pain in others. In order to work towards providing wound care within a framework of culturally competent health care, we need more information on the cultural diversity related to chronic wound pain so that we can develop assessment methods that are sensitive to culturally specific ways of experiencing pain and use this information to develop culturally appropriate treatment goals. This survey is the first step in providing the information necessary to help wound-related pain research include biological, psychological and cultural influences within a model of culturally competent wound care.

Acknowledgements

The research team would like to thank all those patients who took time to complete this questionnaire and all staff across all the countries involved who graciously gave their time. We would also like to acknowledge Rhys Maidment and Paul Heatley for data input and Dr Clio Spanou for her help in Phase I of the study. We would also like to thank Mölnlycke Healthcare for an unrestricted educational grant to support this work.

This chapter was originally published in the *International Wound Journal*: Price P, Fagervik-Morton H, Mudge EJ, *et al* (2008) Dressing-related pain in patients with chronic wounds: an international patient perspective. *International Wound Journal* 2: 159–71. It is republished with kind permission from Wiley-Blackwell.

References

Brennan F, Carr DB, Cousins M (2007) Pain management: a fundamental human right. *Anesth Analg* 105: 205–21

Briggs M, Torra i Bou J (2002) *Pain at wound dressing changes: a guide to management.* EWMA Position Document: *Pain at wound dressing changes.* MEP Ltd, London: 12–17

Charles H (1995) The impact of leg ulcers on patients' quality of life. *Professional Nurse* 10: 571–4

Ebbeskog B, Ekman S-L (2001) Elderly people's experiences. The meaning of living with Venous Leg Ulcer. *EWMA J* 1: 21–3

European Wound Management Association (2002) EWMA Position Document: *Pain at wound dressing changes.* MEP Ltd, London

Franks PJ, Moffatt CJ, Connolly M, *et al* (1994) Community leg ulcer clinics: effect on quality of life. *Phlebology* 9: 83–6

Horn S, Munafo M (1998) *Pain: theory research and intervention.* Open University Press, London

Koral CT, Craig KD (2001) Pain from the perspectives of health psychology and culture. In: Kazarian SS, Evans DR, eds. *Handbook of Cultural Health Psychology.* Academic Press, San Diego

Lindholm C (2007) *Quality of life in patients with leg ulcers and psychological complications.* Atlantio Meetings APT Feridas (Portugese Wound Healing Association) Madeira, 7 December 2007

Melzack R, Wall P (1982) *The Challenge of Pain.* Penguin, Harmondsworth

Moffatt C, Franks P, Hollingworth H (2002) *Understanding wound pain and trauma: an international perspective.* EWMA Position Document: *Pain at wound dressing changes.* MEP Ltd, London: 2–7

Mudge E (2007) Tell me if it hurts: the patient's perspective of wound pain. *Wounds UK* **3**: 6–7

Price P, Harding KG (1996) Measuring health-related quality of life in patients with chronic leg ulcers. *Wounds* **8**: 91–4

Quirino J, Santo V, Quednau T, Martins A, Lima P, Almeida M (2003) Pain in pressure ulcers. *Wounds* **15**: 381–9

Reddy M, Kohr R, Queen D, Keast D, Sibbald RG (2003) Practical treatment of wound pain and trauma: a patient-centered approach. An overview. *Ostomy Wound Management* **49**(4A Suppl): 2–15

Rich A, McLachlan L (2003) How living with a leg ulcer affects people's daily life: a nurse-led study. *J Wound Care* **12**: 51–4

Tu W (1980) A religiophilosophical perspective on pain. In: Kosterlitz HW, Terenius LY, eds. *Pain and Society.* Verlag, Weinheim, Germany: 63–78

Woo K, Sadavoy J, Sidani S, Maunder R, Sibbald RG (2007) *The relationship between anxiety, anticipatory pain, and pain during dressing change in the older population.* CAWC Annual Conference, November 1–4, London, Ontario

World Union of Wound Healing Societies (2004) Principles of best practice: Minimising pain at wound dressing-related procedures. A consensus document. MEP Ltd, London

Chapter 3

Acute and chronic pain in wounds

Andy Roden and Trudie Young

This chapter examines research into the occurrence/incidence, severity and patient descriptions of wound pain, according to different wound types, namely:

- burns
- fungating wounds
- procedural pain and surgical wound pain
- diabetic foot ulcers
- pressure ulcers
- venous leg ulcers.

A literature search was carried out using CINAHL, MEDLINE and the Cochrane Database using the search terms 'wound' and 'pain'; the search was focused by adding 'diabetic foot ulcer', 'burns', 'surgical wound', 'fungating wound', ' pressure ulcer' and 'venous leg ulcer'. All searches were conducted from 2004 to 2008; a total of 120 papers were selected for review. Although some papers did not meet the specific requirements of occurrence/incidence, severity or patient reporting of wound pain, cross-referencing the papers revealed more articles that did fulfil the search criteria. It was decided to link surgical wound pain with incident pain, for example, from iatrogenic sources such as bandaging and debridement, although it was acknowledged that incident pain may be associated with any of the above listed wounds.

The Wound Union of Wound Healing Societies (WUWHS, 2004) describes pain as common in patients with chronic wounds, such as pressure ulcers, leg ulcers and foot ulcers. It is estimated that more than 300,000 people in the UK have chronic pain caused by leg ulcers, and that hundreds of thousands more have pain related to pressure and diabetic foot ulcers (www.news.bbc.co.uk/1/hi/health/4743474. stm). Pain is usually described as existing when the patient says it does (McCaffery and Pasero, 1999). However, it has long been recognised that this is far too simplistic as McCaffery and Beebe (1989) and Camp (1988) noted differences between nurses' and patients' perceptions of the degree of pain.

All wounds have the potential to cause pain, and many factors may exacerbate wound pain such as infection, trauma at dressing changes and poor technique when applying compression therapy (Young, 2007). The pain associated with wounds is not only distressing physically and emotionally, but also impacts further onto the patient's quality of life (Reddy *et al*, 2003).

> *Wound pain is multi-faceted and manifests itself in a combination of chronic persistent pain (caused by the underlying condition) and acute pain (caused by regular dressing changes).*
>
> (Mudge *et al*, 2008, p.21)

The prevalence of wounds within the inpatient and outpatient population was examined in a large study conducted by Srinivasaiah *et al* (2007); they found that the most common wounds were surgical (41.5%), followed by leg and foot ulcers (37.3%) and then pressure ulcers (17.4%). However, figures relating to the incidence of wound pain do vary greatly. For example, estimates for severe or continuous pain in leg ulcers vary between 17–65% (Dallam *et al*, 1995; Ebbeskog and Emami, 1996).

Reporting of pain in different wound types

Burns

The pain of a burn wound may occur in any or all of the three phases associated with burns:

- acute phase, which is often during the initial debridement
- healing phase, which is pain caused by dressing changes
- rehabilitation phase (Summer *et al*, 2007).

The multifaceted nature of burns requires ongoing assessment and flexibility on the part of the practitioner to adapt to patients' pain(s) as they arise (*Chapter 7*).

The complex nature of pain associated with burns has been well documented over many years, yet despite this it remains undertreated (Summer _et al_, 2007). Patterson _et al_ (2006) suggested the reason for this appeared to be a reluctance to prescribe and administer analgesic drugs, especially opioids, because of perceived problems such as overdose and addiction.

Ineffective treatment of pain in the acute phase of burn injury is associated with long-term sequelae such as paraesthesia, dysaesthesia and psychological problems (van Loey and van Son, 2003). Studies of 534 patients with burn injuries suggested that between 71–82% of patients reported paraesthesia in their wounds one year after the initial injury (Khedr _et al_, 1997; Kowalske _et al_, 2001).

Patients' reports of their pain often use language suggestive of a neuropathic element, with terms such as 'pins and needles', 'stabbing', 'burning' or 'shooting' commonly used (Schneider _et al_, 2006).

It should also be remembered that pain insensitivity syndromes such as Riley–Day syndrome, autonomic neuropathy and polyneuropathy as a result of diabetes may render the patient susceptible to burns from trivial sources. Baker _et al_ (2006) reported a case study where full-thickness burns were caused by an electric hand drier, with no pain to the patient.

In addition to assessing the type and severity of the pain, Ratcliff _et al_ (2006) highlighted the importance of other factors relating to paediatric burns, such as itching and post-traumatic stress, which also need to be addressed. They found that the introduction of a burn patient pain protocol incorporating anxiolytics in conjunction with analgesics yielded good results. An interesting observation is that the introduced protocol advocated the use of non-steroidal anti-inflammatory drugs (NSAIDs; e.g. ibuprofen), whereas Tengvall _et al_ (2006) cautioned that NSAIDs should not be used in patients with burns as their antiplatelet effects may increase blood loss and have negative side-effects on renal function.

Fungating wounds

Approximately 5–10% of patients with metastatic cancer will develop a fungating wound (Dowsett, 2002). The rate of malignancy in leg ulceration has been put as high as 4.4 per 100 leg ulcer patients in Australia (Waters _et al_, 2006), although the European figures were lower (Baldursson _et al_, 1993; Hansson and Andersson, 1998). Despite this, Naylor (2001) noted that there have not been any significant surveys of wound pain in this patient group.

The pain of fungating wounds represents a challenge for the practitioner as the pain may result from tissue necrosis, disruption of capillaries and lymph vessels or by compression or infiltration of a nerve by malignant cells (Naylor, 2001). This may manifest itself as sharp, stabbing pain or, if nerves are invaded or compressed, signs of neuropathy, such as allodynia (pain elicited from a light touch) or numbness. The management of fungating wounds is further complicated by issues of odour, exudate, poor self-image and isolation (Mekrut-Barrows, 2006).

The literature on palliative care of patients with fungating wounds is limited. Additionally, integration of palliative care concepts and chronic wound management is challenging (Langemo, 2006) (*Chapter 6*).

Procedural pain and surgical wound pain

Wounds require the application of dressings to protect them; however, the application of bandages, tapes or adhesive dressings may cause pain when being replaced or removed (White, 2008; *Chapter 12*). Moffatt *et al*'s (2002) study suggested dressing removal to be the most painful aspect of the dressing procedure. This is borne out by the findings of Meaume *et al* (2004), who found that 79% of patients experienced moderate to severe pain episodes during dressing change or removal, with between 47–59% experiencing very severe pain in self-evaluation questionnaires.

The Heal Not Hurt campaign (2008; www.healnothurt.co.uk) based upon best practice documents (European Wound Management Association (EWMA), 2002; WUWHS, 2004) emphasised the importance of attempting to reduce procedural pain, e.g. at dressing change. This includes obtaining a detailed pain assessment using a validated assessment tool and assessing the pain between, as well as during dressing changes. The campaign also emphasised the importance of taking patient information before starting the procedure; the results of a small pilot study by Borrie *et al* (2004) supported the value of patient information. They found that in cases where the nurse gave the patients information about the procedure, such as discussing strategies they could use to make it as comfortable as possible, there was a reduced level of pain and/or distress following the intervention.

Recent research appears limited in relation to surgical wound pain, although Melling and Leaper (2006) noted that the postoperative pain associated with hernia repair is an important challenge, and that warming the wound may be beneficial in reducing pain.

Diabetic foot ulcers

Foot ulcers are a significant complication of diabetes mellitus and often precede lower extremity amputation. The most frequent underlying aetiologies are neuropathy, trauma and foot deformity (Armstrong and Lavery, 1998; Frykberg, 2002). The damage to the nerves and vascular supply in the feet and legs result in approximately 4–10% of people with diabetes suffering from chronic ulceration (Ribu and Wahl, 2004). Reiber _et al_ (1998) suggested from epidemiological studies that 2.5% of people with diabetes develop foot ulcers every year, and that 15% may develop a diabetic foot ulcer during their lifetime. The potential impact was discussed by Stillman (2008), who stated that diabetic peripheral neuropathy (present in 60% of people with diabetes and in 80% of people with diabetes and foot ulcers), confers the greatest risk of ulceration. Even after successful management resulting in ulcer healing, the recurrence rate in that patient population is 66% with an amputation rate rising to 12%.

Patients suffering diabetic neuropathy pose a potentially difficult problem for the practitioner as some may feel little or no pain or sensation in the foot, to the extent that they are unaware that further tissue damage may be occurring, such as scalding from hot water (American Diabetes Association, 1999). However, Ribu _et al_'s (2006) data from 127 patients with diabetic foot ulcers attending outpatient clinics found that 75% reported some pain relating to their foot ulcers, with 57% reporting pain on movement; 25% reported no pain at any time. The overall incidence of painful neuropathy is estimated between 10% (Young _et al_, 1993) to nearly 20% (Dyck _et al_, 1993).

Patients' descriptions of their pain associated with diabetic foot ulcers are often associated with other neuropathic conditions, such as 'burning', 'numbing' and 'tingling'. It is interesting to note that chronic pain was significantly more common in diabetic patients compared with a group of non-diabetic control patients (25.2% _vs_ 15.5%, respectively; Chan _et al_, 1990). Chan _et al_ (1990) also reported that up to 25% of people with diabetic foot ulcers had no treatment for pain, although this may be because the areas affected had paraesthesia and therefore were insensate to the patient.

Pressure ulcers

Within the field of pressure ulceration there are few published studies designed solely to capture the prevalence of pain in a pressure ulcer population. However, studies (often qualitative in design) have identified the presence of pain within cohorts of patients with pressure ulcers (Szor and Bourguignon, 1999; Langemo *et al*, 2000; Neil and Munjas, 2000; Fox, 2002; Rastinehad, 2006; Hopkins *et al*, 2006; Spilsbury *et al*, 2007); data have also emerged from quantitative studies or general wound audits (van Rijswijk, 1993; Dallam *et al*, 1995; Hatcliffe and Dawe, 1996; Lindholm *et al*, 1999; Eriksson *et al*, 2000).

One of the first reports of the prevalence of pain in patients with pressure ulcers was published by Dallam *et al* in 1995. This study was undertaken in an acute care setting where over half of the patients ($n = 78$; 59%) with pressure ulcers ranging from superficial to deep-tissue damage reported pain of some type. However, more pain was experienced by those with deeper and more severe ulceration; this relationship was also reported in later studies (Szor and Bourguignon, 1999; Lindholm *et al*, 1999; Eriksson *et al*, 2000). Subsequent figures for the prevalence of pain in patients with pressure ulcers range from 37.1% (Lindholm *et al*, 1999) to 91% (Spilsbury *et al*, 2007).

More detail on the severity of the pain reported by patients with pressure ulcers was provided by Szor and Bourguignon (1999). Their study reported on 32 patients with pressure ulcers (grades 2–4, $n = 28$), of whom 87.5% experienced pain at dressing change; the pain was described as mild, discomforting, distressing, horrible or excruciating. Quirino *et al* (2003) found burning to be the most common term used to describe pressure ulcer pain. This is also reported by Neil and Munjas (2000), who included stinging, sharp, stabbing and tingling as adjectives that portrayed the pain. In a study of 151 patients, Hatcliffe and Dawe (1996) reported that 30% had mild pain, 12% moderate pain and 7% severe pain. Langemo *et al* (2000) described the extreme pain that patients associate with pressure ulceration. Conversely, in a study of 119 patients with 153 pressure ulcers, 21 patients (37.5%) were said to be pain free; however, data relating to the severity of these pressure ulcers was not presented (van Rijswijk, 1993).

Although dressing change has been identified as a time when pain is experienced (Hopkins *et al*, 2006), it is also reported to be present at rest (Szor and Bourguignon, 1999; Eriksson *et al*, 2000; Quirino *et al*, 2003). The timing of the pain occurrence can vary, with it changing from day to day and hour to hour (Quirino *et al*, 2003; Spilsbury *et al*, 2007).

Rastinehad (2006) refers to the actions of healthcare personnel and treatment interventions as painful experiences. The pain of debridement is cited as causing great physical and emotional distress to patients (Neil and Munjas, 2000). Treatment options have been described as easing the pain (hydrocolloid dressings) and also causing the pain (static air replacement mattresses) (Szor and Bourguignon, 1999). Recent studies reaffirm this notion, when pressure-relieving equipment was found to exacerbate pressure ulcer pain and a hoist was found to cause ulcers (Hopkins _et al_, 2006; Spilsbury _et al_, 2007).

When trying to establish the prevalence of pain in pressure ulcers, a major difficulty is separating the pain of the pressure ulcer and the pain of other associated conditions often found in patients with pressure ulcers, such as arthritis, infection, ischaemia and carcinoma (Reddy _et al_, 2003). In a paediatric population, 73.8% of the children had pain that was not associated with their pressure ulcers (Willock and Harris, 2007). An additional complexity is establishing the presence and severity of the pain, with the previous studies all using a variety of methods and tools to accomplish this. However, Clark (2002) highlights the fact that individuals with pressure ulcers may be unable to complete the assessments, even with the assistance of trained data collectors, thus having an effect on the ability to quantify the human costs of pressure ulcers. A recent, systematic review acknowledged that there are no published statistics on the incidence of pain in pressure ulcers, but noted that in published prevalence studies the figures were higher when a validated measurement tool had been used (Girouard _et al_, 2008).

Venous leg ulcers

The prevalence of pain in patients with venous leg ulceration has been reported in various publications spanning the past 10 years. Hofman _et al_ (1997) reported that 64% (n = 60) of patients experienced ulcer pain, but a lower prevalence of 58% (n = 35) was identified in a Canadian community study (Nemeth _et al_, 2003). In a more recent study (Jones _et al_, 2006), 35% (n = 67) of patients had mild pain, 37% (n = 70) had moderate to overwhelming pain and 28% (n = 53) had no pain at all. Pain was the main presenting problem for 85% of patients surveyed in an outpatient population (141 patients) having leg ulceration of varying aetiology.

Patients' attitudes to wound pain appear to be one of inevitability, with an expectation that pain will accompany leg ulceration (Krasner,

1998; Mudge *et al*, 2006). The ulcer pain appears to develop from something that acts as a prompt to seek medical help, to an all-encompassing focus of daily life (Husband, 2001; Briggs *et al*, 2006).

The terminology used by patients to describe their ulcer pain gives some indication of its severity.

Sore, burning, shooting, red hot needles, very bad, nagging toothache (Walshe, 1995).

Aching, annoying, burning, dull, hot poker, sticking pins in, hot, hurting, nagging, nerve pain, sharp, shooting, sick-in-the-stomach pain, stabbing, sticky, stinging, throbbing, tingling, uncomfortable (Krasner, 1998).

Aching, stabbing, throbbing, burning, sharp, tender (Noonan and Burge, 1998).

Throbbing, sharp, itchy, tender (Charles *et al*, 2002).

Nagging toothache, sharp, burning, dull, niggly, gnawing, stabbing (Hareendran *et al*, 2005).

Burning, deep pain, red hot poker, throbbing, itching (Mudge *et al*, 2008).

In addition, effective descriptors, e.g. exhausting, sickening and cruel indicate the impact that the ulcer pain has on the individual (Noonan and Burge, 1998). Interestingly, non-intravenous drug users described their ulcer pain in a more stoic fashion than their counterparts who were using intravenous drugs, with the latter describing their ulcer pain as being of crippling intensity (Palfreyman *et al*, 2006).

The main site of the pain is usually in the ulcer bed. However, Hofman *et al* (1997) identified three distinct locations for the pain: within the ulcer, around the ulcer, and elsewhere in the leg. Additionally, patients often have pain in more than one site. Pain in the area surrounding the ulcer is frequently linked to maceration from wound exudate. The ulcer pain can be a constant feature or occur intermittently (Jones *et al*, 2006). The level of the pain experienced can also vary in intensity throughout the day (Mudge *et al*, 2008).

A key consequence of ulcer pain is sleep disturbance (Walshe, 1995; Hofman *et al*, 1997; Krasner, 1998; Noonan and Burge, 1998;

Bentley, 2006; Stevens, 2006; Briggs, 2006), and patients have described being in a constant state of tiredness (Mudge _et al_, 2008). Mobility is also adversely affected by the pain, resulting in reduced and limited movement. The ulcer pain is often aggravated by standing, which further restricts the individual in their activities of daily living (Walshe, 1995; Hofman _et al_, 1997; Krasner, 1998; Noonan and Burge, 1998; Bentley, 2006; Stevens, 2006). Conversely, resting with legs elevated caused pain for certain individuals (Hofman _et al_, 1997). Swelling of the legs, which can be associated with immobility, was another factor that equated with an increase in ulcer pain (Krasner, 1998).

Healthcare interventions should hopefully be associated with pain reduction, although this is not always the outcome. Patients reported pain and, conversely, pain relief during wound cleansing (Briggs and Closs, 2006). In the same study, patients reported ulcer pain instigated by wound dressings, including hydrogels, low-adherent dressings, foams, hydrofibre and antimicrobial dressings. The whole dressing procedure can stimulate various aspects of pain: anticipatory pain is experienced before dressing change; and removal and reapplication of a dressing can be painful or provide pain relief, especially if this signals the end of the procedure (Mudge _et al_, 2008). However, for most patients the procedure continues with the subsequent application of compression therapy, which is associated with a temporary or constant increase in ulcer pain. The pain may result in the individual being unable to tolerate the treatment (Husband, 2001; Briggs and Closs, 2006). Conversely, a reduction in pain was identified in a randomised, controlled trial that used short-stretch compression therapy (Charles _et al_, 2002). A second study that focused on care delivery systems found a statistically significant reduction in pain for individuals receiving care in a leg club model (Edwards _et al_, 2005).

The physical aspect of ulcer pain is only one dimension. Depression and anxiety was present in 53% ($n = 102$) of patients with chronic venous ulceration (Jones _et al_, 2006). One of the symptoms that was associated with the depression and anxiety was pain.

Conclusion

It is well established in the literature that pain is present across a myriad of wound types, although exact prevalence figures are at times absent. These statistics are further complicated by the different patient populations sampled and the varying size between the samples, with the research methodology often dictating the size of the population examined (Khedr *et al*, 1997; Kowalske *et al*, 2001; Mudge *et al*, 2008). Further impediments to the data collection process are the presence of neuropathy and the inability of the individual to communicate his or her pain experience effectively (Dyck *et al*, 1993; Young *et al*, 1993; Baker *et al*, 2006; Stillman, 2008). However, for those who are able to describe their pain, the terminology used has similarities across different wound types (Chan *et al*, 1990; Krasner, 1998; Schneider *et al*, 2006).

A current theme across most wound types is the lack of effective pain management. This appears to be underpinned by an imbalance between taking sufficient medication and a willingness to avoid any side-effects, often resulting in subtherapeutic analgesic treatment (Patterson *et al*, 2006). This is frequently confounded by the provision of mixed messages from the many healthcare personnel involved with a patient with a wound (Grocott *et al*, 2008). Analgesic regimens appear to be enhanced by additional interventions, such as the use of protocols, providing adequate information and warming the wound (Borrie *et al,* 2004; Melling and Leaper, 2006; Ratcliff *et al,* 2006).

A common occurrence that appears across most wound types is the prevalence of procedural pain (Eriksson *et al*, 2000; Neil and Munjas, 2000; Husband, 2001; Meaume *et al*, 2004; Hopkins *et al*, 2006; Rastinehad, 2006; Spilsbury *et al*, 2007). This reinforces the views of healthcare professionals who perceive dressing changes as a painful event (EWMA, 2002; Price *et al*, 2008; *Chapter 2*).

The complexity of wound pain cannot be underestimated, with the pain experience having a multitude of dimensions. Patients vividly describe the physical, social and psychological components of wound pain and the impact that this has on their daily lives (Jones *et al,* 2006; Mekrut-Barrows, 2006).

References

American Diabetes Association (1999) *Consensus Development Conference on Diabetic Foot Wound Care* http://care.diabetesjournals.org/cgi/reprint/22/8/1354.pdf [accessed 25 September 2008]

Armstrong DG, Lavery LA (1998) Evidence-based options for off-loading diabetic wounds. *Clin Podiatr Med Surg* 15: 95–104

Baker R, Smith M, Cussons P (2006) The insensate burn: pain insensitivity syndrome. *Burns* 32(2): 255–7

Baldursson B, Sigurgeirsson B, Lindelof B (1993) Leg ulcers and squamous cell carcinoma: an epidemiological study and a review of the literature. _Acta Derm Venerol_ **73**: 171–4

Bentley J (2006) Improving quality of life in venous leg ulceration: a case study. _Br J Nurs_ **15**: 4–8, 19

Borrie MG, Goettl L, Campbell K, _et al_ (2004) Educational intervention in the management of acute procedure-related wound pain: a pilot study. _J Wound Care_ **13**(5): 187–90

Briggs M (2006) quoted in Elliott J, ed. 'My ulcers left me in constant pain'. http://news.bbc.co.uk/1/hi/health/4743474.stm [accessed 25 September 2008]

Briggs M, Closs SJ (2006) Patients' perceptions of the impact of treatments and products on their experience of leg ulcer pain. _J Wound Care_ **15**(8): 333–7

Briggs M, Flemming K, Closs SJ (2006) _Living with Leg Ulceration: A Meta-synthesis of Qualitative Research_. The 2006 International Nursing Research Conference. Royal College of Nursing, London

Camp LD (1988) A comparison of nurses' recorded assessments of pain with perceptions of pain as described by cancer patients. _Cancer Nurs_ **11**(4): 237–43

Chan AW, Macfarlane IA, Bowsher D, _et al_ (1990) Chronic pain in patients with diabetes mellitus: comparison with a non-diabetic population. _Pain Clin_ **3**: 147–59

Charles H, Callicot C, Mathurin D, _et al_ (2002) Randomised, comparative study of three primary dressings for the treatment of venous ulcers. _Br J Community Nurs_ **7**(suppl): 48–54

Clark M (2002) Pressure ulcers and quality of life. _Nurs Standard_ **16**(22): 74–80

Dallam L, Smyth C, Jackson BS, Krinsky R, _et al_ (1995) Pressure ulcer pain: assessment and quantification. _J Wound Ostomy Continence Nurs_ **22**(5): 211–15, 217–18

Dowsett C (2002) The role of the nurse in wound bed preparation. _Nurs Standard_ **16**: 69–72, 74, 76

Dyck PJ, Kratz KM, Karnes JZ, _et al_ (1993) The prevalence by staged severity of various types of diabetic neuropathy, retinopathy and nephropathy in a population-based cohort: the Rochester Diabetic Neuropathy Study. _Neurology_ **43**: 817–24

Ebbeskog B, Emami A (1996) Older patients' experience of dressing changes on venous leg ulcers: more than just a docile patient. _J Clin Nurs_ **14**(10): 1223–31

Edwards H, Courtney M, Finlayson K, _et al_ (2005) Improved healing rates for chronic venous leg ulcers: pilot study results from a randomised controlled trial of a community nursing intervention. *Int J Nurs Pract* **11**(4): 169–76

Eriksson E, Asko-Seljavaara S, Hietanen H (2000) Prevalence and characteristics of pressure ulcers. A one-day patient population in a Finnish city. *Clin Nurse Specialist* **14**(3): 119–25

European Wound Management Association (2002) EWMA Position Document: *Pain at wound dressing changes*. MEP Ltd, London

Fox C (2002) Living with a pressure ulcer: a descriptive study of patients' experiences. *J Wound Care* **11**(6): 10–22

Frykberg RG (2002) Diabetic foot ulcers: pathogenesis and management. *Am Fam Physician* **66**(9): 1655–62

Girouard K, Harrison MB, Vandenkerkof E (2008) The symptom of pain with pressure ulcers: a review of the literature. *Ostomy Wound Management* **54**(5): 30–40, 42

Grocott P, Roden A, Hofman D, McManus J (2008) Debate: How should we approach pain management in wound care? *Wounds UK* **4**(3): 105–9

Hansson C, Andersson E (1998) Malignant skin lesions on the legs and feet at a dermatological leg ulcer clinic during five years. *Acta Derm Venereol* **78**: 147–8

Hareendran A, Bradbury A, Budd J, *et al* (2005) Measuring the impact of venous leg ulcers on quality of life. *J Wound Care* **14**(2): 53–7

Hatcliffe S, Dawe R (1996) Clinical audit. Monitoring pressure sores in a palliative care setting. *Int J Palliative Nurs* **2**: 182–6

Heal Not Hurt campaign (2008) http://www.healnothurt.co.uk Mölnlycke Health Care [accessed 25 September 2008]

Hofman D, Ryan TJ, Arnold F, *et al* (1997) Pain in venous leg ulcers. *J Wound Care* **6**(5): 222–4

Hopkins A, Dealey C, Bale S, Defloor T, Worboys F (2006) Patient stories of living with a pressure ulcer. *J Adv Nurs* **56**(4): 345–53

Husband LL (2001) Venous ulceration: the pattern of pain and paradox. *Clin Effectiveness Nurs* **5**: 35–40

Jones V, Grey JE, Harding KG (2006) Wound dressings. *Br Med J* **332**(7544): 777–80

Khedr EM, Khedr T, El-Oteify A, *et al* (1997) Peripheral neuropathy in burn patients. *Burns* **23**: 579–83

Kowalske K, Holavanahali R, Helm P, *et al* (2001) Neuropathy after burn injury. *J Burn Care Rehab* **22**: 353–7

Krasner D (1998) Pain and venous ulcers: theme and stories about their impact on quality of life. *Ostomy Wound Management* **44**(9): 38–9

Langemo DK (2006) When the goal is palliative care. *Adv Skin Wound Care*

19(3): 148–54

Langemo DK, Melland H, Hanson D, Olson B, Hunter S (2000) The lived experience of having a pressure ulcer: a qualitative analysis. _Adv Skin Wound Care_ **13**(5) 225–35

Lindholm C, Bergsten A, Berglund E (1999) Chronic wounds and nursing care. _J Wound Care_ **8**(1): 5–10

McCaffery M, Beebe A (1989) Giving narcotics for pain. _Nursing_ **19**(10): 161–5

McCaffery M, Pasero C (1999) Assessment: underlying complexities, misconceptions and practical tools. In: McCaffery M, Pasero CL, eds. _Pain: Clinical Manual._ 2nd edn. Mosby, St Louis: 35–102

Meaume S, Téot L, Lazareth I, Martini J, Bohbot S (2004) The importance of pain reduction through dressing selection in routine wound management: the MAPP study. _J Wound Care_ **13**(10): 409–13

Melling AC, Leaper DJ (2006) Warming, its impact on pain and wound healing after hernia surgery: a preliminary study. _J Wound Care_ **15**(3): 104–8

Mekrut-Barrows C (2006) Softening the pain of cancer-related wounds. _Ostomy Wound Management_ **52**(9): 12–13

Moffatt CJ, Franks PJ, Hollingworth H (2002) Understanding wound pain and trauma: an international perspective. EWMA Position Document: _Pain at wound dressing changes._ MEP Ltd, London: 2–7

Mudge E, Holloway S, Simmonds W, et al (2006) Living with venous leg. ulceration: issues concerning adherence. _Br J Nurs_ **15**(21): 1166–71

Mudge E, Spanou C, Price P (2008) A focus group study into patients' perception of chronic wound pain. _Wounds UK_ **4**(2) http://www. wounds-uk.com/cgi-bin/journal_view_abstract.cgi?articleid=0402_focus [accessed 25 September 2008]

Naylor W (2001) Assessment and management of pain in fungating wounds. _Br J Nurs_ **10**(22 suppl): S33–6

Neil JA, Munjas BA (2000) Living with a chronic wound: the voices of sufferers. _Ostomy Wound Management_ **46**(5): 28–34, 36–8

Nemeth KA, Graham ID, Harrison MB (2003) Pain with venous leg ulcers: point prevalence study at three time periods. _Adv Skin Wound Care_ **16**(5): 260–7

Noonan L, Burge S (1998) Venous leg ulcers: is pain a problem? _Phlebology_ **13**: 14–19

Palfreyman SJ, Nelson EA, Lochiel R, et al (2006) Dressings for healing venous leg ulcers. _Cochrane Database Syst Rev_ (3) CD001103

Patterson DR, Tininenko MA, Ptacek JT (2006) Pain during burn hospitalization predicts long-term outcome. _J Burn Care Res_ **27**(5): 719–26

Price P, Fagervik-Morton H, Mudge EJ, et al (2008) Dressing-related pain in patients with chronic wounds: an international patient perspective. *Int Wound J* 2: 159–71

Quirino J, Santos VLC, Quednau TJP, Martins, *et al* (2003). Pain in pressure ulcers. *Wounds* 15: 381–9

Rastinehad D (2006) Pressure ulcer pain. *J Wound Ostomy Continence Nurs* 33(3): 252–7

Ratcliff SL, Brown A, Rosenberg M, *et al* (2006) The effectiveness of a pain and anxiety protocol to treat the acute pediatric burn patient. *Burns* 32: 554–62

Reddy M, Keast D, Fowler E, Sibbald RG (2003) Pain in pressure ulcers. *Ostomy Wound Management* 49(4): 30–5

Reiber GE, Lipsky BA, Gibbons GW (1998) The burden of diabetic foot ulcers. *Am J Surg* 176: 5S–10S

Ribu L, Rustoen T, Birkeland K, *et al* (2006) The prevalence and occurrence of diabetic foot ulcer pain and its impact on health-related quality of life. *J Pain* 7: 290–9

Ribu L, Wahl A (2004) Living with diabetic foot ulcers: a life of fear, restrictions, and pain. *Ostomy/Wound Management* 50(2): 57–67

Schneider JC, Harris NL, El Shami A, *et al* (2006) A descriptive review of neuropathic-like pain after burn injury. *J Burn Care Res* 27(4): 524–8

Spilsbury K, Nelson EA, Cullum C, *et al* (2007) Pressure ulcers and their treatment and effects on quality of life: hospital inpatient perspectives. *J Adv Nurs* 57: 494–504

Srinivasaiah N, Dugdall H, Barrett S, *et al* (2007) A point prevalence survey of wounds in north-east England. *J Wound Care* 16(10): 413–16, 418–19

Stevens H (2006) The impact of venous ulcer pain: what can the patient teach us? *Br J Community Nurs* 11(12 Suppl): S27–S30

Stillman RM (2008) *Wound Care*. http://www.emedicine.com/MED/topic2754.htm [accessed 25 September 2008]

Summer GJ, Puntillo KA, Miaskowski C, *et al* (2007) Burn injury pain: the continuing challenge. *J Pain* 8(7): 533–48

Szor JK, Bourguignon C (1999) Description of pressure ulcer pain at rest and at dressing change. *J Wound Ostomy Continence Nurs* 26(3): 115–20

Tengvall OM, Bjornhagen VC, Lindholm C, *et al* (2006) Differences in pain patterns for infected and non-infected patients with burn injuries. *Pain Manage Nurs* 7(4): 176–82 (p178)

van Loey NE, MJ van Son (2003) Psychopathology and psychological problems in patients with burn scars: epidemiology and management. *Am J Clin Dermatol* 4(4): 245–72

van Rijswijk L (1993) Full-thickness pressure ulcers: patient and wound healing characteristics. *Decubitus* 6: 16–21 van Rijswijk L, Lyder CH (2005) Pressure ulcer prevention and care: implementing the revised guidance to surveyors for long-term care facilities. *Ostomy Wound Manage* **April** (suppl): S7–S19

Walshe C (1995) Living with a venous leg ulcer: a descriptive study of patients' experiences. *J Adv Nurs* **22**: 1092–100

Waters J, Latta A, Hartley A, *et al* (2006) Malignancy and leg ulceration in a community-based leg ulcer clinic in New Zealand. *J Wound Care* **17**(6): 264–6

White R (2008) A multinational survey of the assessment of pain when removing dressings. *Wounds UK* **4**(1): 14–24

Willock J, Harris C, Harrison J, *et al* (2007) Identifying the characteristics of children with pressure ulcers. *Nurs Times* **101**(11): 40–3

World Union of Wound Healing Societies (2004) Principles of best practice: Minimising pain at wound dressing-related procedures. A consensus document. London: MEP Ltd

Young MJ, Boulton AJ, Maclead AF, *et al* (1993) A multicentre study of the prevalence of diabetic peripheral neuropathy in the United Kingdom hospital clinic population. *Diabetologia* **36**: 150–4

Young T (2007) Assessment of wound pain: overview and a new initiative. *Br J Nurs* **16**(8): 456–61

Chapter 4

Neuropathic pain

Tzvetanka Ivanova-Stoilova

The International Association of the Study of Pain (IASP) defines neuropathic pain as a type of chronic pain initiated or caused by primary lesion or dysfunction of the peripheral or central nervous system (Meskey and Bogduk, 1994). Patients do not usually present with identifiable neurological disease but with symptoms, therefore a dysfunction can be difficult to prove (Aggarwal *et al*, 2006). The clinical course of neuropathic pain does not have a defined circuitry, it can be of long or even lifetime duration and has a profound impact on a person's quality of life.

Epidemiology

A recent survey of chronic pain in Europe found that one in five adults report chronic pain (Breivik *et al*, 2006). In previous studies of the whole population the prevalence of neuropathic pain has been found to be 2–4 % (Bowsher, 1991). In a very recent study, Bouhassira *et al* (2008) found a prevalence of chronic pain in the general population in France of 31.7%; 6.9% of which had neuropathic characteristics. The high prevalence of neuropathic pain was concluded by the use of screening tool (DN 4 questionaire, Bouhassira *et al*, 2005) to detect neuropathic signs and symptoms. In Austria, Gustoff *et al* (2008) found a 3.3% prevalence of neuropathic pain, with higher prevalence of 26% in adults aged 41–50 years. Many patients are treated for neuropathic pain in primary care in the United Kingdom (Hall *et al*, 2006). In people who have suffered from diabetes for 15–20 years, 25–50% are affected by diabetic polyneuropathy (Quattrini and Tesfaye, 2003; Vinik, 2004). With an increasing elderly population, the prevalence of neuropathic pain (for example, postherpetic neuralgia) is expected to rise with a corresponding demand for healthcare resources (Schmader, 2002).

Aetiology

Neuropathic pain can be caused by many conditions (*Table 4.1*).

Clinical characteristics of neuropathic pain

Neuropathic pain can be recognised both by clinical signs (what the physician finds on examination) and symptoms (what the patient reports). The pain can be described as:

Table 4.1: Conditions that cause neuropathic pain	
Central nervous system	poststroke pain
Idiopathic conditions	peripheral neuropathies
Infection	herpes zoster, human immunodeficiency virus (HIV)
Inflammatory conditions	multiple sclerosis (MS)
Malignancy	tumour invasion, metatastic disease, cancer treatment
Metabolic conditions	diabetes, hypothyroidism, hyperthyroidism
Myofascial entrapment	piriformis syndrome, anterior scalene syndrome
Orthopaedic conditions	radiculitis, radiculopahty, cord compression
Postsurgical pain	post herniotomy, post mastectomy, stump pain, phantom pain
Toxic	alcohol, heavy metal poisoning, cytostatics
Trauma	spinal cord injury, brachial plexus avulsion, complex regional pain syndrome type I
Unknown conditions	restless leg syndrome
Vascular conditions	migraine, cluster headache, trigeminal neuralgia, peripheral vascular disease

- burning
- stinging
- pins and needles sensation
- lancinating (a sensation of cutting, piercing, or stabbing)
- hot poker
- ice cold.

The hallmarks of neuropathic pain are abnormal sensations such as:

- hyperalgesia: an increased response to a normally painful stimulus (e.g. pin prick)
- allodynia: pain evoked by an innocuous stimulus (touch, pressure, brush, warmth) (*Figure 4.1*)
- static: painful response simply from a light brush
- dynamic: pain as a result of pressure.

Patients with neuropahtic pain may also have:

- hyperpathia: an unpleasant sensation with slow onset and increasing severity and distribution area
- hypoaesthesia: a reduced response to touch, pin prick, temperature
- dysaesthesia: an unpleasant abnormal sensation.

In neuropathic pain, the clinical signs and symptoms can be positive or negative, coming from the sensory, motor and autonomic nervous system (*Table 4.2*).

Clinical symptoms of neuropathic pain have the following range:

- continuous or intermittent
- spontaneous (non-stimulus provoked) or evoked (provoked by stimulus)
- superficial or deep
- burning or cold
- sharp or dull
- paroxysmal (shooting, lancinating)
- itching.

Neuropathic pain has an ill-defined circuitry, duration and response to treatment. It can last long after a surgical operation scar has healed or the rash from a shingles infection has disappeared. It does not usually

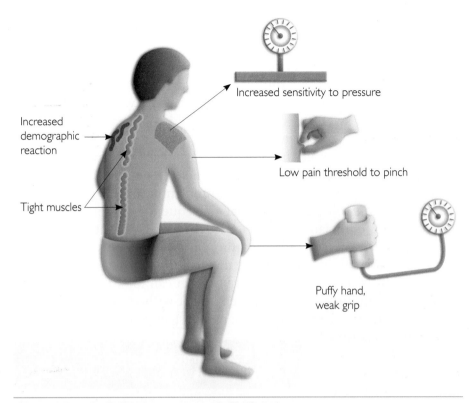

Increased sensitivity to pressure

Increased demographic reaction

Low pain threshold to pinch

Tight muscles

Puffy hand, weak grip

Figure 4.1: Clinical presentation of allodynia

respond to simple painkillers or anti-inflammatory drugs. The pain may appear in bursts, unprovoked by body position, active or passive movement. Patients with neuropathic pain with the same aetiology (for example, postherpetic neuralgia) can have different responses to the same pharmacological agent (antidepressant, anticonvulsant or topical agent). Frequently, the side-effects of the pharmacological agents are intolerable and need to be discontinued or reduced, with suboptimal control of symptoms. The severity and complexity of patients' symptoms vary with time and should be frequently evaluated. In cases of severe pain (e.g. complex regional pain syndrome type 1 or 2, trigeminal neuralgia), the initial treatment plan may need to be comprehensive (pharmacological, injection treatment, physical rehabilitation, psychological treatment, social support and addressing issues of safety in the home and work place), so that symptoms are quickly put under control. Thereafter, the therapeutic effect can be maintained with pharmacological treatment only. People suffering from neuropathic pain may have movement disorders (weak hand grip, difficulty in weight-bearing), making activities of daily living and work difficult to perform. Some patients are distressed by the experience of distorted body image — a sensation of expansion of the affected limb when there is no visible change in size. Temperature of the affected body part can be perceived differently compared with temperature on palpation (feet feel cold, but on palpation they are warm). Autonomic changes such as swelling, redness, shiny skin, increased or reduced sweating vary and improve with control of the pain. They are not accompanied by systemic inflammatory response (no change in white cell count, C-reactive protein, erythrocyte sedimentation rate).

Neuropathic pain can have a profound impact on a patient's life, with serious psychological and social consequences. Often, the patient as well as the clinician feels frustrated by the fact that, in contrast to musculoskeletal pain, neuropathic pain cannot be controlled by modification of activity — it may be there all the time or come in bursts with no identifiable trigger. The area of pain can look normal and the patient's description of symptoms may meet with scepticism from the clinician which inevitably makes the patient feel that his complaint has not been taken seriously. The fact that it is not always a symptom of an identifiable neurological condition can be depressing for the patient, as he may assume that nobody knows what is wrong with him and subsequently the prescribed therapy may not meet with his confidence and compliance.

It is imporant to explain to the patient that the pain does not come from the site itself, but from the nerves supplying this site. It is often more severe at night, leading to sleep disturbance and

Table 4.2: Neuropathic signs and symptoms	
Negative	**Positive**
Sensory	
hypoaesthesia	para and dysaestheia
hypoalgesia	hyperalgesia, allodynia
anosmia	hyperosmia
amaurosis	photopsia
deafness	tinnitus
Motor	
paresis, paralysis	myotonia, fasciculations
Autonomic	
vasodilation	vasoconstriction
anhydrosis	hyperhydrosis
piloerection deficit	piloerection

deprivation, and subsequent daytime fatigue and exhaustion (Edwards _et al_, 2008). Low mood, lack of control, frustration, fear and anger compound the course of neuropathic pain. Depression is the most frequent psychiatric comorbidity which augments the painful state, making it harder to treat (Argoff 2007; Wise _et al_, 2007).

Diagnostic tools

Quantitative sensory testing and electrophysiological studies can be used to help diagnose neuropathic pain. However, due to time constraints or lack of equipment, this is not routine practice. Several assessment tools have been developed to help the clinician recognise neuropathic pain. Two of the most recent ones are based on patient reports of symptoms and clinical examination. These are the Leads Assessment of Neuropathic Signs and Symptoms scale (LANSS) (Bennett, 2001) and the more recent DN 4 questionnaire (Bouhassira _et al_, 2005).

The LANSS scale will identify neuropathic pain on a score of > 12 and the DN 4 questionnaire on a score equalling > 4 out of 10.

Pathophysiology

Neuropathic pain is caused by changes in the structure and function of the peripheral and central nervous system. These changes can explain some of its symptoms and diversity in patients with one and the same aetiology. Neuropathic pain can be an expression of a myriad of increased/reduced levels of neurotransmitters, activation of channels, erratic cross-talk between neurones, deficient anti-nociceptive system, structural reorganisation of neurones in the spinal cord and in the brain (_Figure 4.2_). For example, postherpetic neuralgia pain can in one patient be hyperaesthetic, and in another, dysaesthetic.

Neuropathic pain mechanisms at the periphery

There is a nociceptor sensitisation with increased sensory output. The peripheral non-myelinated C-fibres (slow pain transmission) and myelinated Aδ (conveying the fast pain) widen their receptive field and show reduced stimulation threshold to thermal and mechanical

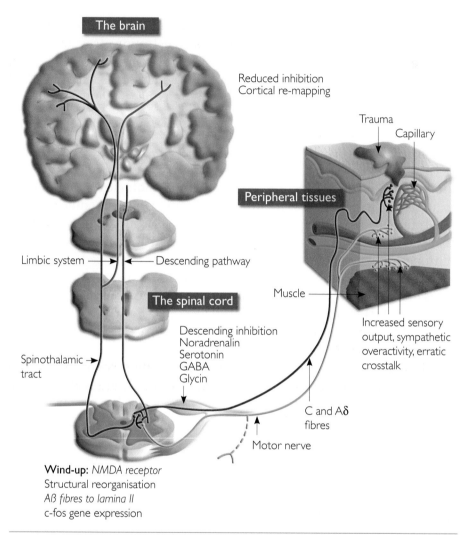

Figure 4.2: Main pathophysiological changes in neuropathic pain

stimuli. Clustering of sodium channels at the injured nerve endings causes ectopic impulses in axons and the dorsal root ganglion with erratic cross-talk between neurons. The autonomic nervous system can show signs of sympathetic over activity (Byers and Bonica, 2001). This structural and functional reorganisation is accountable for the hallmark symptom of hyperalgesia.

Neuronal re-modelling and hypersensitisation at the spinal cord

The spinal cord has got an important role in the modification of pain transmission. In acute pain, the stimulation of Aβ-fibres (conveying mechanical stimulus perception) reduces or stops the pain transmitted by C and Aδ-fibres, therefore closing the gate of pain transmission from peripheral tissues to the brain (Gate control theory of pain) (Wall and Melzack, 1965).

In neuropathic pain, there is anatomical reorganisation of Aβ-fibres with their growth into lamina (_Lamina gelatinosa_), instead of synapse in the deeper layers of the spinal cord (lamina IV). Therefore, the stimulation of Aβ-fibres elicits pain, in contrast to closing the gate in acute pain. This phenomena explains the other hallmark of neuropathic pain, allodynia.

The persistence of pain long after tissue healing has taken place has been explained by the 'wind-up' phenomenon caused by activation of the N-methyl d-aspartate receptor (NMDAR) (Jenssen _et al_, 2003). In acute pain, this receptor is inactive by Mg^{++} ion plug. However, with continuing neurotransmitter bombardment (glutamate, aspartate), the Mg block is removed and the receptor is activated allowing continuing influx of Ca^{++} ions, irrespective of the lack of further stimulation from the periphery (Jensen _et al_, 2003).

The expression of receptors and neurotransmitters can be fixed in the genome by _cis-fos_ genes (Morgado and Tavares, 2007), and is accountable for the persisting symptoms long after tissue healing has occurred.

The anti-nociceptive system

Pain perception is modified and reduced by the central anti-nociceptive system which operates by noradrenalin and serotonin release and production of inhibitory neurotransmitters (GABA, glycin). In chronic pain, including neuropathic pain, the anti-nociceptive system can be deficient. As a result, inter neuronal inhibitory transmission is reduced in the peripheral nerve endings, spinal cord and brain. The release of endorphins and encephalins stimulates the production of inhibitory neurotransmitters, which modify the pain impulse (Fields and Basbam, 1994).

The brain

The human brain is the central station of pain perception with cortical representation of body zones as expressed in the sensory post central gyrus.

However, in conditions where there is a lack of peripheral input (e.g. after limb amputation), there is restructuring and shifting of the representation of body zones (Ramachandran's theory of adult brain plasticity) (Ramachandran and Rogers-Ramachandran, 2000).

In limb amputation, phantom pain can be a result of deafferentation with activation of central neuronal network and re-mapping of body zones on the postcentral gyrus, with resultant distressing and disabling pain. The brain plasticity explains the telescoping of the phantoms with time and the provocation of phantom pain on stimulation of adjacent body zone (shaving the face can provoke upper limb phantom pain). Further, morphometric analyses of the brain in different chronic pain conditions (i.e. phantom limb pain, chronic back pain, fibromyalgia, chronic headache) resulted in a loss of grey matter in the cingulated cortex, the orbito-frontal cortex, insula and the dorsal pons, therefore indicating the role of structural and functional reorganisation of the central nervous system in the perpetuation of pain when there is no longer input from the periphery (May, 2008).

Treatment of neuropathic pain

Treatment of neuropathic pain is a challenging and difficult task. The clinician needs to consider carefully which medicine to prescribe and how best to use it, while the patient will also need to comply with the medication and lifestyle advice given.

It is important to remember that neuropahtic pain can be a feature of an underlying condition like diabetes, vitamin deficiency, intoxication or tumour, and the patient should be investigated to establish the cause of the symptoms. Furthermore, correction of the underlying cause can reverse or stop its progression (e.g tight glycaemic control for diabetic neuropathy, vitamin B12 in pernicious anaemia, thyroxin supplement for hypothyroidism).

Correction of the underlying condition may be non-urgent (alcohol-related, idiopathic, postsurgical), urgent (trauma, infection, tumour, nerve root compression) or an emergency (spinal cord compression or *cauda equina* syndrome [CES]).

The clinician is frequently challenged by questions, such as:

Is it a dysfunction or lesion?
How long will it last?

Will it ever go away?
Which medication shall I try and what shall I do next if it is
not helping?
How long shall I try to treat the patient before I ask for help from a
specialist in pain medicine?

Neuropathic pain needs to be evaluated within the context of the pathophysiology of the underlying condition, or the progression of the disease _per se_. For example, radiculopathic pain may not be the solo cause of a patient's pain five years since the initial onset, as his symptoms may be due to subsequent development of spinal stenosis with resultant spinal claudication.

The swelling that accompanies wounds on limbs can impair the blood supply of the perineurium of the bypassing nerves, giving rise to neuropathic pain from the common peroneal nerve at the knee, or the sural nerve at the lateral aspect of the ankle. This can outlast the nociceptive pain due to tissue destruction or inflammation around the wound. On the other hand, treating neuropathic pain reduces the sympathetic output, improves microcirculation and speeds the healing process.

Identification of symptoms and signs of neuropathic pain can prompt the underlying pathophysiological mechanisms (Jensen and Baron, 2003). For example, a case of postherpetic neuralgia with unpleasant sensations and skin numbness (dysaesthetic pain) will be treated differently compared to a case with skin hypersensitivity (hyperaesthetic pain), as the former involves mainly central sensitisation, and the latter, a peripheral sensitisation.

At present, the principles of treatment of neuropathic pain are aetiological, pathophysiological and according to signs and symptoms. The choice of drugs or their combination and stepwise inclusion in the treatment algorithm will be presented in the light of the current evidence of their efficacy.

Pharmacological management

The complex pathophysiological mechanisms and the numerous molecular targets in neuropathic pain has prompted treatment with a wide range of pharmacological agents (_Chapter 8_) (Mcquay, 1996; Sindrup and Jenssen, 1999; Galer _et al_, 2002; Rowbotham _et al_, 2004; Finnerup _et al_, 2005; Goldstein _et al_, 2005; Moulin _et al_, 2007):

- antidepressants
- anticonvulsants
- benzodiazepines
- antiarrythmics
- local anaesthetics
- weak opioids
- topical preparations.

In clinical trials, drug efficacy and safety has been measured by two numbers: the number needed to treat (NNT), which is the number of patients treated for one of them to achieve a 50% reduction in severity of pain (Cook and Sackett, 1995); and the number needed to harm (NNH), i.e. the number of patients treated for one of them to discontinue a clinical trial due to side-effects.

Only a few of the drugs currently used for treating neuropathic pain have been licensed, namely:

Anticonvulsants:
- carbamazepine for trigeminal neuralgia, mechanism of action — blockade of Na^+ channels
- gabapentine for neuropathic pain
- pregabalin for peripheral neuropathic pain, mechanism of action — blockade of subunit of neuronal Ca^{++} channel.

Anti-parkinson drugs:
- mirapexin for restless legs syndrome, mechanism of action — unknown.

Antidepressants:
- tricyclic antidepressants — amitriptyline, imipramine — enhance the noradrenalin release from the anti-nociceptive system
- serotonin-noradrenalin reuptake inhibitors (SNRIs)
- duloxetine for diabetic neuropathy, mechanism of action — increased inhibition via inhibited reuptake of adrenaline and serotonin.

Topical:
- capsaicin for neuropathic pain; mechanism of action — depleting the stores of substance P in the periphery and spinal cord
- lidocaine 5% medicated plaster for postherpetic neuralgia — blockade of peripheral nerve Na^+ channels and interrupting pain transmission.

Sindrup and Jensen (1999) compared the efficacy of pharmacological agents and their mechanism of action and, more recently, Finnerup *et al* (2005) proposed an algorithm for the treatment of neuropathic pain based on existing evidence of efficacy.

Table 4.3 shows the NNT and NNH for the most commonly used pharmacological agents for painful diabetic neuropathy (DN), while *Table 4.4* shows the NNT for agents used to treat postherpetic neuralgia (PN).

From the above evidence it is clear that neuropathic pain is a challenging issue and that, at its best, a single modal treatment can alleviate symptoms by 50% in approximately 1/3 of patients treated for the condition (as one can calculate from the NNT). It is imperative to communicate to the patient that the therapeutic options will alleviate rather than abolish symptoms, which may persist for a long time. Pharmacological agents needed to treat this type of pain also have their own side-effects (*Table 4.3*), these may develop slowly or be apparent at the onset of treatment resulting in discontinuation before a useful therapeutic effect has been achieved. It is important to explain the most common side-effects and how to overcome them — such as drowsiness at the onset of treatment with gabapentinoids (slow titration), constipation with opioids (laxatives taken regularly).

Table 4.3: Commonly used pharmacological agents for painful diabetic neuropathy (DN)

DN	NNT	NNH
Imipramine/amitriptyline	2.4	14.7
Carbamazepine	3.3	21.7
Tramadol	3.4	
Gabapentin	3.7	17.8
Pregabalin	4.2	11.7
Capsaicin	5.9	
Selective serotonin reuptake inhibitor (SSRI)	6.7	
Venlafaxine	4.6	
Mexiletine	10	

(Rowbotham, 2004; Goldstein *et al*, 2005)

Table 4.4: NNT for agents used for treatment of PN

PHN	NNT	NNH
Oxycodone	2.5	
Morphine	2.7	
Tramadol	4.8	7.9
Gabapentin	5.1	
Pregabalin	4.2	
Topical capsaicin	6.7	11.5
Topical lidocaine	4.4	

(Finnerup *et al*, 2005)

Table 4.5: Common side-effects of pharmacological agents

Tricyclic antidepressants	dry mouth, constipation, urinary retention, arrythmias, sedation
Anticonvulsants	sedation, dizziness, memory disturbance, ataxia, peripheral oedema, weight gain, blurred vision
Opioids	nausea, itching, sedation, respiratory depression, constipation, urinary retention, addiction
Tramadol	nausea, sedation, constipation, convulsions, orthostatic hypotension
SNRIs	hypertension, tachycardia, sedation, nausea, suicide ideation

Drug administration regimes can involve dose titration. For example, gabapentine needs to be started as a single dose taken at bedtime (100 or 300 mg), and gradually increased over one week to one three times/ day. Dose ranges can be diverse (from 300 mg to 1800 mg/day), and the titration of the dose should match the clinical response and be the most beneficial to and tolerated by the patient. Pregabalin, which is another gabapentinoid, is started at an initial dose of 75 mg twice/daily (b.d.), and can be titrated to 150 mg b.d and further increased to 300 mg b.d. according to clinical response. In contrast to gabapentin, it has got linear pharmacokinetics, so the higher the dose, the better the analgesic effect.

Table 4.6 shows guidelines of management of neuropathic pain on the basis of existing evidence (Attal *et al*, 2006).

The British Pain Society and the Pain Committee of the Royal College of General Practitioners have produced the following guidelines for management of neuropathic pain in primary care:

Treating neuropathic pain: A primary care three-month plan, BPS and PC of RCGP, January 2008		
Non-focal		**Focal**
First month	TCA/anticonvulsant	5% lidocaine plaster
Second month	Combine both +/- tramadol	
Third month	Strong opioids for severe pain — modified release or trans- dermal formulation	
Refer to specialist at any stage if diagnosis is unclear and the patient does not respond to treatment		

Non-pharmacological treatments

Psychological treatments

As chronic, non-malignant pain is a biopsychosocial event which has a profound impact on a person's life, psychological treatments play an important role in conjunction with the pharmacological and other non-pharmacological therapies (*Chapter 9*). These involve cognitive behavioural treatment (CBT), relaxation, positive imaging, individual and group counselling (Williams *et al*, 1993). Such therapies can help patients and their families cope better with a long-term condition that can have a severe negative impact on quality of life. Since 2004, the author's clinic have been running educational seminars for patients with diabetic neuropathies and their healthcare professionals, which have improved motivation, compliance with medication, and exercise (Ivanova-Stoilova *et al*, 2007).

Interventional procedures

Within a comprehensive treatment plan, interventional procedures with local anaesthetic/depo steroid mixtures aim to break the vicious

Table 4.6: Treatment plans for each drug

Drug	Daily dose	Frequency	Maximum daily dose	Titration	Comments
Tricyclic antidepressants					
Amitriptyline	10–25 mg	od	150 mg	Increase by 10–25 mg weekly	Muscarinic effects, sedation
Nortriptyline	10–25 mg	od	75 mg	Increase by 10–25 mg weekly	Less sedating
Anticonvulsants					
Gabapentin	300 mg	tds	1800 mg	Increase by 100–300 mg daily to maximum 1800 mg	Somnolence, ataxia, cognitive impairment, oedema
Pregabalin	150 mg	bd	600 mg	Increase by 25 mg to effect	May be effective if no response to gabapentin
Carbamazepine	200 mg	bd–qds	800 mg	Increase slowly to effect	First line for trigeminal neuralgia, ataxia, sedation
SSRIs/SNRIs					
Duloxetine	60 mg	od	120 mg		Sedation, hypertension, suicide ideation
Venlafaxine	37.5–75 mg	od	200 mg	Increase by 37.5 mg weekly	Gradual withdrawal
Weak opioids					
Tramadol	50–150 mg	tds–qds	400 mg	50–100 mg tds–qds	Nausea, dizziness, constipation
Strong opioids					
Morphine	20–120 mg	bd–slow release	Increase weekly		Sedation, nausea, constipation, respiratory depression, addiction
Oxycodone	20–80 mg	bd–slow release	Increase weekly	400 mg	May be effective where morphine not tolerated
Topical agents					
Capsaicin	0.025%	qds	Use sparingly over unbroken skin	0.075%	Burning, stinging, do not apply heat, do not bandage
Lidocaine plaster	5%	12 hours on, 12 hours off		Three plasters at a time	Not waterproof, very low systemic absorption

circle of pain, spasm, and inactivity. In the author's clinic, treatments with peripheral nerve blocks, trigger point injections, fluoroscopically guided piriformis and iliopsoas muscle blocks (*Figures 4.3a, b*), lumbar sympathetic blockade, neuraxial blocks and dorsal root ganglion blocks for segmental pain have been performed (Ivanova-Stoilova, 2007). Neuromodulation and neuro-destructive procedures include:

- radiofrequency and pulsed radiofrequency (*Figure 4.4*)
- denervation of painful scars, neuromas
- treatment of segmental pain.

The implantation of a spinal cord stimulator has been found to reduce symptoms in patients with complex regional pain syndrome type 1, as well as painful diabetic neuropathies (Sundaraj *et al*, 2005)

There is less evidence to show that acupuncture, transcutaneous electrical nerve stimulation (TENS), and alternative therapies help (Abuiash, 1998; Brunelli, 2004).

In treating phantom limb and stump pain, positive imaging, mirror exercises, early fitting with functional prosthetic limbs, and a Faraday cage shield (Farablock; a special cloth made up of cotton + metal fibres which forms a faraday cage and guards off positive ions from atmosphere when put on the stump) have been used. Mirror therapy has been beneficial in reducing the pain and increasing movement in the affected limb and is related to reducing or reversing the changes by the cortical reorganisation of the body zone (Brodie, 2007; Schwarzer, 2007) (*Figure 4.5*).

Physical therapy

The main aim of physical therapy is to relieve pain, restore muscle flexibility and strength, improve a joint's torque, and enhance the healing process. Physical rehabilitation is important following a pain relief intervention, for example, ilipsoas muscle-stretching, ankle exercises, core stability exercises and so on.

The treatment of patients with neuropathic pain necessitates not only quantitative and qualitative evaluation of the pain type, but also functional assessment that can serve an objective measure of patients' progress. We use the 'timed up and go' test (Podsiadlo, 1991) to measure mobility of diabetic patients with painful neuropathies. This test is easy to perform and can be used by the patient himself

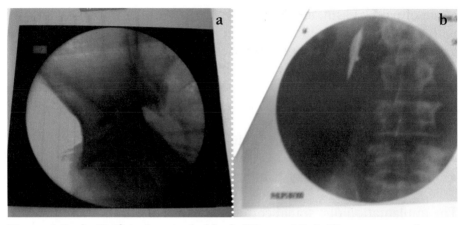

Figure 4.3a, b: Piriformis muscle block (Figure 4.3a); Iliopsoas muscle block (Figure 4.3b)

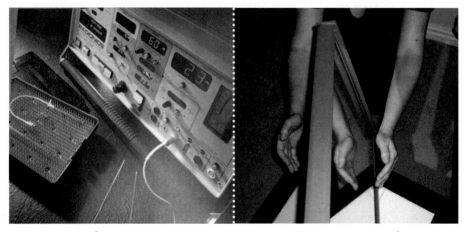

Figure 4.4: Radionics radiofrequency generator

Figure 4.5: Mirror exercises for complex regional pain sydrome type 1, (the painful hand is behind the mirror)

to monitor progress in mobility, encourage motivation and be an objective indicator of success as a result of comprehensive treatment (Ivanova-Stoilova *et al*, 2007).

It should be remembered that patients with neuropathic pain can present with a myriad of accompanying comorbidities and, in the event of failure of pharmacological therapies, a comprehensive assessment of all presenting pain syndromes is necessary. In our diabetic polyneuropahty pain clinic, an assessment of 52 patients with intractable pain showed that 80% of all patients had accompanying musculoskeletal pain: 10% had non-reconstructable peripheral vascular disease; 10% had myogenic neuropathy pain-piriformis and iliopsoas syndrome; and 25% had other neuropathies (Ivanova-Stoilova _et al_, 2007). Very often, an individual patient will present with several neuropathies and musculoskeletal pain.

Treatment response can be complicated by metabolic state (morbid obesity), cardiovascular problems (peripheral vascular disease, central post-stroke pain), and iatrogenic conditions (statin therapy for hyper-cholesterolaemia, cytotoxics). It is therefore important that the whole physical and pharmacological background of the patient is considered to achieve the best possible clinical outcome.

References

Aggarwal VR, McBeth J, Zakrzewska JM, Lunt M, Macfarlane GJ (2006) The epidemiology of chronic syndromes that are frequently unexplained: do they have common associated factors? _Int J Epidemiol_ 35: 468–76

Argoff CE (2007) The coexistence of neuropathic pain, sleep and psychiatric disorders: a novel treatment approach. _Clin J Pain_ 23(1): 15–22

Attal N, Cruccu G, Haanpaa P, Jensen TS, Nurmikko T, Sampaio C, _et al_ (2006) EFNS guidelines on pharmacological treatment of neuropathic pain. _Euro J Neurol_ 13: 1153–69

Bennett MI (2001) The LANSS Pain Scale: the Leeds assessment of neuropathic symptoms and signs. _Pain_ 92: 147–5

Bouhassira D, Lanteri-Minet M, Attal N, Laurent B, Touboul C (2008) Prevalence of chronic pain with neuropathic characteristics in the general population. _Pain_ 136: 380–7

Bouhassira D, Attal N, Alchaar H, Boureau F, Bruxelle J, Cvunin G, _et al_ (2005) Comparison of pain syndromes associated with nervous or somatic lesions and development of a new pain diagnostic questionnaire (DN4). _Pain_ 114: 29–36

Bowsher D (1991) Neurogenic pain syndromes and their management. _Br Med Bull_ 47(3): 644–66

Breivik H, Colett B, Ventafridda V, Cohen R, Gallacher D (2006) Survey of chronic pain in Europe: prevalence, impact on daily life and treatment. _Eur J Pain_ 10: 287–333

British Pain Society (2005) _Recommendations for the appropriate use of opioids for persistent non-cancer pain: A Consensus statement prepared on behalf of the British Pain Society, the Royal College of Anaesthetists,_ the Royal College of General Practitioner and the Royal College of Psychiatrists. British Pain Society, London

Brodie EE, Whyte A, Niven CA (2007) Analgesia through the looking-glass? A randomized controlled trial investigating the effect of viewing of virtual limb upon phantom limb pain, sensation and movement. *Eur J Pain* 11(4): 428–36

Brunelli B, Gorson KC (2004) The use of complementary and alternative medicines by patients with peripheral neuropathy. *J Neurol Sci* 21 (1–2): 59–66

Byers MR, Bonica JJ (2001) Peripheral pain mechanisms and nociceptor plasticity. In: Loeser JD, ed. *Bonica's Management of Pain.* 3rd edn. Lippincott Williams & Wilkins, Philadelphia: 26–72

Cook RJ, Sackett DL (1995) The number needed to treat: a clinically useful measure of treatment effect. *Br Med J* 310: 452–4

Edwards RR, Almeida DM, Klick B, Haythornthwaite JA, Smith MT (2008) Duration of sleep contributes to next-day pain report in the general population. *Pain* 137: 202–7

Fields Hl, Basbam AL (1994) Central nervous system mechanisms of pain modulation. In: Wall PD, Melzack R, eds. *Textbook of Pain.* 3rd edn. Churchill Livingstone, New York: 243–57

Finnerup NB, Otto M, McQuay HJ, *et al* (2005) Algorithm for neuropathic pain treatment: An evidence-based proposal. *Pain* 118: 289–305

Galer BS, Jensen MP, Ma T, *et al* (2002) The lidocaine patch 5% treats all neuropathic pain qualities: results of a randomized, double-blind, vehicle-controlled, 3-week efficacy study with use of the neuropathic pain scale. *Clin J Pain* 18(5): 297–301

Goldstein DJ, Lu Y, Detke MJ, Lee TC, Iyengar S (2005) Duloxetine v.s. placebo in patients with painful diabetic polyneuropathy. *Pain* 116: 109–18

Gustoff B, Dorner T, Likar R, *et al* (2008) Prevalence of self-reported neuropathic pain amd impact on quality of life: a prospective representative survey. *Acta Anaesthesiol Scand* 51(1): 132–6

Hall GC, Caroll D, Parry D, McQuay HJ (2006) Epidemiology and treatment of neuropathic pain: The UK primary care perspective. *Pain* 122(1–2): 156–62

Ivanova-Stoilova TM, Donne P, Jones L, Wilson E, Wartan S (2007) Persisting pain in patients with diabetes — new diagnostic and therapeutic approaches from our new diabetic polyneuropathy pain clinic. BPS, ASM Glasgow 2007; Poster abstracts PC29

Ivanova-Stoilova TM, Wartan S (2007) *The role of local anaesthetic blocks in improving clinical outcome for patients with diabetic neuropathies and* _intractable pain_. 3rd International Forum on Pain Medicine, Montreal 2007; Program and abstract book: 124

Jensen TS, Baron R (2003) Translation of symptoms and signs into mechanisms in neuropathic pain. _Pain_ **102**(1–2): 1–8

May A (2008) Chronic pain may change the structure of the brain. Review. _Pain_ **137**: 7–13

McQuay HJ, Tramer M, Nye BA, _et al_ (1996) A systematic review of antidepressants in neuropathic pain. _Pain_ **68** : 217–27

Merskey H, Bogduk N (1994) _Classification of Chronic Pain: Descriptions of Chronic Pain Syndromes and Definitions of Pain Terms_. 2nd edn. IASP Press, Seattle

Morgado C, Tavares I (2007) C-fos expression at the spinal dorsal horn of streptozocin-induced diabetic rats. _Diabetes Metab Res Rev_ **23**(8): 644–52

Quattrini C, Tesfaye S (2003) Understanding the impact of painful diabetic neuropathy. _Diabetes Meta Res Rev_ **19S**: S2–S8

Ramachandran VS, Rogers-Ramachandran D (2000) Phantom limbs and neural plasticity. _Arch Neurol_ **57**(3): 317–20

Rowbotham MC, Goli V, Kinz NR, Lei D (2004) Venlaflaxine extended release in the treatment of painful diabetic neuropathy: A double-blind, placebo-controlled study. _Pain_ **113**: 697–706

Royal College of Anaesthetists and The Pain Society (2003) Pain Management services. Good Practice, May 2003

Sindrup SH, Jensen TS (1999) Efficacy of pharmacological treatments of neuropathic pain: an update and effect related to mechanism of drug action. _Pain_ **83**: 389–400

Schmader KE (2002) Epidemiology and impact on quality of life of postherpetic neuralgia and painful diabetic neuropathy. _Clin J Pain_ **18**: 350–4

Schwarzer A, Glaudo S, Zenz M, Maier C (2007) Mirror feed-back — new method for treatment of neuropathic pain. _Dtsch Med Wochen schr_ **132**(41): 2159–62

Sundaraj SR, Johnstone C, Noore F, _et al_ (2005) Spinal cord stimulation: a seven-year audit. _J Clin Neurosci_ **12**(3): 264–70

Vinik AI, Mehrabyan A (2004) Diabetic neuropathies. _Med Clin N Am_ **88**: 947–99

Williams AC, Nicholas MK, Richardson PH, _et al_ (1993) Evaluation of cognitive behavioural programme for rehabilitating patients with chronic pain. _Br J Gen Pract_ **43**: 513–8

Wise TN, Fishbain DA, Holder-Perkins V (2007) Painful physical symptoms in depression: a clinical challenge. _Pain Med_ **8** Suppl 2: S75–82

Chapter 5

Pain in paediatric wound care

Jacqueline Denyer

Paediatric wound management occurs throughout many specialties, including neonatal care, elective surgery, trauma and chronic conditions. Whether the wound is a single event, with anticipated uneventful healing without recurrence, or forms part of a long-term chronic condition, the emphasis on pain management must be paramount.

Over recent years there have been vast technical advances in the care and management of acute and chronic paediatric conditions. However, knowledge and evidence base in the management of paediatric wound care is far behind that of the adult population. Relatively few wound care products have been studied in the neonatal and paediatric groups, which are bounded by ethical restraints in carrying out research in this age range. It is not unusual for skin care practice to be based on institutional or individual preference (Baharestani, 2007).

This chapter considers pain management of both acute and chronic wounds in relation to neonates and children. Wherever possible, pain should be assessed using good communication between the child, his or her carers and professionals within the relevant multidisciplinary team (Howard *et al*, 2008). Where effective pain management is complex and difficult to achieve, the team should include a consultant paediatric anaesthetist and a paediatric pharmacist.

Pain in neonatal wound care

Types of wounds commonly occurring within the neonatal period include epidermal stripping, napkin excoriation, chemical burns, thermal injury, pressure ulcers and extravasation injuries (Wound Academy, Mölnlycke Health Care, 2005).

Surgical wounds result from the correction of congenital abnormalities or complications of prematurity, such as necrotising enterocolitis. Wounds resulting directly from genetic defects, such as epidermolysis bullosa or ichthyosis, require long-term adaptations to handling and dressing techniques (Denyer, 2006).

It has been demonstrated that neonates potentially feel more pain than older infants, and that early exposure to pain may have long-term effects on perception of pain and behaviour (Anand, 1998; Johnson _et al_, 1999).

Pain assessment tools for acute procedural pain in neonates include the Premature Infant Pain Profile (PIPP; Jonsdottir and Kristjansdottir, 2005). While forming an important part of the pain assessment process, tools should be used in conjunction with views of parents and other carers; environmental factors and individual characteristics should also be given consideration.

General recommendations in neonatal pain management include the use of sucrose for brief procedures and permitting the mother to breast feed throughout the procedure. A great deal of research has been carried out to show the effectiveness of sucrose in offering temporary analgesia to reduce stress associated with invasive or distressing procedures (Stevens _et al_, 2004). Sucrose should be used with caution in infants with necrotising enterocolitis and with those who are intubated. The preparation should be administered 1–2 minutes before the procedure in the form of 0.1 ml sucrose solution to the tongue or buccal mucosa. The dose can be repeated when the procedure starts and repeated every two minutes if required (Morash and Fowler, 2004; Hunt and Peters, 2007).

Use of oral sucrose in association with venepuncture, removal of a chest drain, urine sampling by catheterisation and lumbar puncture is well documented, but little information is available about its use in the management of wound pain. In the author's experience, sucrose supplements traditional pain relief for dressing changes and is beneficial on its own for short dressing changes. Again, in the author's experience, allowing the mother to breast feed or bottle feed throughout a dressing change greatly increases comfort during the procedure.

Principles of paediatric wound pain management

Pain assessment

Pain assessment forms the essential basis of ensuring pain is both prevented and relieved (Howard, 2003). Accuracy of pain assessment is dependent on the age of the child and his or her cognitive ability (Wound Academy, Mölnlycke Health Care, 2004). No single measure for pain assessment can be recommended across all children. Where possible, management of wound pain should include both non-pharmacological and pharmacological strategies.

Self-reporting of pain by children is considered to be the most important factor in pain assessment. However, this can be difficult for some if there is impaired cognitive ability or for those in a young age group (Breau *et al*, 2001). Therefore, in addition to self-reporting, assessment should be used in conjunction with physiological signs and observations of behavioural characteristics.

There is a vast array of paediatric pain assessment tools available. Self-report tools for assessing postoperative and procedural pain include:

- *FACES pain scale* (Wong and Baker, 1988) for 3–18-year olds
- *Visual analogue and numerical rating scales* for children ≥8 years (Stinson *et al*, 2006)
- *Pieces of Hurt tool* (Hester, 1979) for 3–8-year olds
- *The multiple size poker chip tool* (MSPCT; St-Laurent-Gagnon *et al*, 1999) for 4–6-year-olds (see Howard *et al*, 2008 for a review of assessment tools).

Physiological measures such as heart rate changes in the older child can be reliably used in conjunction with self-reporting of pain to form an assessment. It should be noted that respiratory rate, heart rate and blood pressure are not reliable indicators of pain in neonates, infants and very young children.

Families, nursing staff and play therapists can reduce anxiety by good preparation. It is often beneficial for children to receive psychological preparation before painful dressing changes in a non-emergency situation.

The environment

Children with traumatic wounds will generally be seen initially in the accident and emergency (A&E) department. This in itself is frequently busy with many distressed patients and relatives in evidence. Ideally, there should be a designated paediatric department or area in a general A&E department that is child-friendly. Dressing changes may thereafter be performed in the ward environment, and older children can be given the choice of having the dressing changed at their bedside or in a treatment room. Many children prefer dressings to be changed in their own home by community nurses as this removes the fear that additional procedures, such as going to theatre, will be sprung

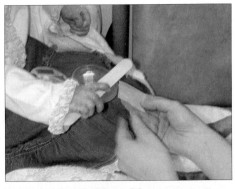

Figure 5.1: Children like to assist in their wound management

upon them. Attention should be given to privacy, particularly for older children and adolescents as they may not wish to see the wound; screening should therefore be available.

Exposure of the wound to air can cause additional pain, so speed of the dressing change is important. Fans should be turned off and the room kept warm. If there is prior knowledge of the wound, templates can be made and dressings pre-cut. Rather than waiting for other professionals to see the wound, photographs can be taken (following permission from the child and parents) for later review.

If wound swabs for microbiology are required, rather than applying a dry swab, it may be appropriate to moisten the swab to reduce the risk of pain when the wound is swabbed (author's observation). Children often prefer to remove and sometimes apply their own dressings themselves or may request their parents to do this following training; this is frequently the case in those suffering from chronic wounds.

Selection of dressing

Although there is a wide knowledge of the benefits from using atraumatic wound dressings among healthcare professionals, in the author's experience selection of dressing material is not always appropriate because suitable dressings are not readily available. This often occurs when there is an urgent need for dressings; for example, when an infant is born with severe epidermolysis bullosa suffering from extensive skin loss. Cost of dressings is often quoted as a reason for selection, but in reality the consequence of a longer healing time is more expensive both in monetary terms and the distress to the child and family.

If the first dressing change is well managed with the selection of an atraumatic dressing (Meaume *et al*, 2004; White, 2005), with appropriate adequate pain relief given and with the procedure taking place in a non-threatening environment, the child is less likely to have anticipatory fear regarding future procedures. Choice of a secondary dressing, where required, is equally important to avoid trauma resulting from adherence of this to the peri-wound skin or to the primary dressing. Consideration should also be given to retention of the dressing and its anticipated removal. Children may prefer retention garments rather than wrap-around or tubular bandages. Where possible, select dressings that can remain in place for several days. If necessary for reasons such as odour or exudate management, the secondary dressing can be changed more frequently while the primary dressing remains *in situ*.

Application of topical antimicrobials such as ointments and honey preparations may cause stinging (Molan, 2001). Even though this is generally transient it is unacceptable in paediatric care, especially in a young child who does not have the ability to recognise that the pain is of short duration. Where the use of such products is desirable, a small area should be tested with the product initially and selection changed if stinging results. Older children can make the decision whether to receive the product or not, following appropriate analgesia. Infection greatly increases wound pain and should be treated promptly, either with topical antimicrobial preparations or with antibiotics (oral or intravenous).

Children with chronic wounds often find bathing painful, as the water can sting the wounds on contact. They may not be able to tolerate all their wounds being exposed at any one time because this can be too painful, make handling difficult and have a negative impact on their body image (author's experience). The bio-burden can be reduced by cleansing the wound and applying the correct antimicrobial preparation or dressing. Where odour is problematic, honey has proved to be effective management.

Adherence of a dressing or clothing to the wound and/or surrounding skin is extremely painful and can potentially lead to an extremely traumatic experience such as skin stripping (Cutting, 2008). The adherent material can often be soaked off or worked free using copious amounts of 50% liquid : 50% white, soft paraffin. In the author's experience, a silicone medical adhesive remover is the most successful in releasing the dressing or clothing without pain or trauma (Mather and Denyer, 2008).

The preferred approach is to avoid wound-related trauma and pain wherever possible. To a degree, this can be achieved by judicious use of atraumatic dressings. For example, in a multicentre study (Morris *et al*, 2008) different types of paediatric wounds/skin injuries were dressed for six weeks' healing using soft silicone dressings with Safetac® technology (Mepilex® Border Lite, Mölnlycke Health Care). Levels of trauma were assessed: healing of the wounds/skin injuries; condition of the surrounding skin; and performance of the dressing in terms of exudate handling, conformability, ease of use, ease of removal and patient comfort.

The results showed that the mean pain severity scores were statistically significantly lower at the first dressing change than at baseline ($P \leq 0.003$). The low pain severity scores compared favourably with those reported in the published literature for other dressing types and pain-relieving strategies. Over 99.5% of the dressing changes were reported to be atraumatic. Over half (55.6%) of the wounds healed within the study period (mean 14.5 days, range 4–42 days), the mean proportion of viable tissue at the final visit (99.5%) was statistically significantly higher than at baseline (90.7%; $P=0.01$) and the proportion of patients exhibiting healthy/intact skin around their wounds increased from 75% at baseline to 91.6% at final visit. No dressing-related adverse events were reported.

Repair of lacerations

Tissue adhesives are generally quicker to apply. For deeper or higher tension lacerations, topical anaesthetic preparations are less painful to apply than injected lidocaine. Where topical anaesthetics are not available or injected lidocaine desirable, this can be buffered with sodium bicarbonate to reduce pain. Hair apposition techniques are less painful than suturing for scalp lacerations and avoid the need for additional distress following shaving (Howard *et al*, 2008).

Dressing changes in a child with burns

Children with burns require repeated changes of dressings; some of these may be changed under general anaesthesia. This is particularly applicable to the initial dressing changes and may be continued thereafter if the child remains distressed. A combination of pharmacological and non-pharmacological therapies should be employed to achieve optimal pain relief (*Chapter 9*) (Laterjet, 2002).

Management of children with chronic wounds

The older child should be involved in the choice of dressing and timing of dressing changes. Despite the longevity of the wound or wounds, consideration must still be given to pain assessment as pain can be variable. Children who are constantly in fear of pain suffer additional anxieties and anticipatory fear (Acton, 2007). Other factors such as pain from other sources in children with complex medical conditions must be considered within the pain assessment.

Children with chronic wounds should have doses of analgesia reviewed regularly and increased in case of tolerance or in line with weight gain.

Neuropathic pain is often a feature in those with chronic wounds. The best management of pain is achieved using a combination of pharmacological and non-pharmacological measures.

Blister management

Blisters may need to be lanced in order to stop them from spreading and causing additional tissue damage. Some children find this procedure to be painful and distressing. In the author's experience, using a cooling spray immediately before lancing the blister reduces pain and leads to a reduction in anticipatory fear.

Pain management at dressing changes

Pharmacology

Paediatric pain regimens comprise local anaesthetics, opioids, non-steroidal anti-inflammatory drugs (NSAIDs) and paracetamol (*Chapter 8*). Ketamine is a dissociative anaesthetic with analgesic properties used to provide systemic or neuraxial analgesia. Inhaled nitrous oxide is helpful for painful procedures and has a role to play in managing pain from dressing changes (Howard *et al*, 2008).

Local anaesthetics

Local anaesthetics are used before repair of lacerations and before minor surgical procedures. Additional analgesia, distraction or nitrous oxide may also be required. Local anaesthetics are not recommended for the management of wounds > 8 cm. The preparations need to be applied for up to 30 minutes before the procedure, which may cause a raised level of anxiety.

Opioids

Opioids are the most powerful group of analgesics and are widely used in the management of painful wounds. Commonly prescribed opioids for children for management of wound pain include morphine, tramadol and fentanyl:

- *Morphine* is the most widely used opioid in children and can be given via many routes. Following surgery or acute trauma, morphine can be given parenterally by continuous or intermittent infusion. For routine dressing changes, morphine is generally given orally 30–60 minutes before the procedure.
- *Tramadol* is increasingly used in children and is proven to be effective against mild to moderate pain. It produces fewer adverse side effects, such as respiratory depression and constipation, than other opioids.
- *Fentanyl* is a potent opioid analgesic. It has a rapid onset of short duration and is therefore useful in the management of children with chronic wounds who require dressing changes before going to school. Fentanyl can be given via the transmucosal route in the form of a lozenge, thus eliminating the need for administration before a dressing change.

NSAIDs

NSAIDs are effective in the management of mild to moderate pain in children. They work more efficiently in combination with paracetamol. Paracetamol is used for the treatment of mild pain. However, when used in conjunction with NSAIDs or a weak opioid, it is successful in managing moderate pain.

Ketamine

Ketamine is an anaesthetic agent given by oral administration, intravenous injection or intravenous infusion. It produces dissociative anaesthesia with amnesia and an altered state of consciousness. It can be associated with hallucinations. Ketamine should be considered in the management of children undergoing prospective painful procedures such as dressing changes following burns or trauma (Rauch, 1998).

Nitrous oxide

Nitrous oxide is a weak, anaesthetic gas with analgesic properties used for analgesia during dressing changes. It is suitable for children over five years who demonstrate the ability to self-administrate by operating the demand valve by means of a mask or mouthpiece (Bruce and Franck, 2000). In the author's experience, nitrous oxide is not suitable in children with long-term chronic wounds, such as those with epidermolysis bullosa, as they expect this to be available at every dressing change and prolonged use may lead to megaloblastic changes in bone marrow.

Anxiolytic medication

Children who undergo multiple dressing changes often develop an anticipatory fear of the procedure. Anxiety can begin as the day of the dressing change approaches. An anxiolytic medication such as midazolam can be given in conjunction with appropriate pain relief to break this cycle. It should be noted that midazolam may prevent the child from exhibiting signs of pain and must always be given with analgesia.

Management of neuropathic pain

Chronic wound pain may be partly neuropathic in origin and may be partially opioid resistant. Treatment with low-dose amitriptyline or with gabapentin is often helpful (Watterson and Denyer, 2006).

Topical pharmacological preparations

Topical morphine has proven to be effective in managing wound pain in paediatrics. Morphine sulphate (10 mg) is mixed with hydrogel (15 ml) and applied either directly to the wound bed or spread onto the dressing, depending on the child's preference (Watterson *et al*, 2004). The concentration of morphine can be increased until optimal pain relief is achieved.

Dressings impregnated with ibuprofen provide topical pain relief and have proven helpful for the management of painful wounds. However, these are not licensed for children < 12 years.

Non-pharmacological pain relief in paediatric wound management

Research on the effects of distraction therapies in reducing burn procedural pain demonstrates that anticipation of pain increases pain intensity, which can be decreased by diverting the child's attention (Laterjet, 2002).

Psychological interventions for procedural pain are aimed at reducing pain and distress through the modulation of thought and behaviour. Techniques effective in procedural pain management in paediatrics include distraction, guided imagery and hypnosis (Uman *et al*, 2006):

- **Distraction** is the easiest technique to apply, and diverts attention away from the procedure and its related pain. It includes watching films, playing computer games or talking about a favourite topic.
- **Guided imagery** is a therapeutic technique that allows two people to communicate on a reality that one of them has chosen to construe through the process of imaging (Whitaker, 2003). Unlike hypnosis, guided imagery focuses on imaging rather than responsiveness to suggestion (Syrjala and Abrams, 1996).
- *Hypnosis* is a state of heightened awareness and focused attention. This enhances susceptibility and receptiveness to ideas.

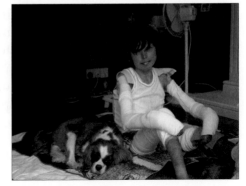

Figure 5.2: Children with life-long dressing requirements find comfort in unorthodox sources such as family pets

Where children require long-term wound management, it is important to introduce these techniques at an early age in order for the child to be receptive to them.

Conclusion

Management of paediatric wound pain is complex and must be specific to the individual. Effective management involves input from a multidisciplinary team and can be achieved through careful dressing selection, a child-friendly environment and a combination of pharmacological and non-pharmacological therapies.

References

Acton C (2007) The holistic management of chronic wound pain. *Wounds UK* **3**(1): 61–9

Anand KJS (1998) Clinical importance of pain and stress in pre-term newborn infants. *Biol Neonate* **73**: 1–9

Baharestani MM (2007) An overview of neonatal and paediatric wound care knowledge and considerations. *Ostomy Wound Management* **53**(6): 34–55

Breau LM, Camfield C, McGrath PJ, Rosmus C, Finley GA (2001) Measuring pain accurately in children with cognitive impairments: refinement of a caregiver scale. *J Paediatr* **138**(5): 721–7

Bruce E, Franck L (2000) Self-administered nitrous oxide (Entonox) for the management of procedural pain. *Paediatr Nurs* **12**: 15–19

Cutting KF (2008) Impact of adhesive surgical tape and wound dressings on the skin, with reference to skin stripping. *J Wound Care* **17**(4): 157–62

Denyer J (2006) Epidermolysis bullosa. In: White RJ, Denyer J, eds. *Paediatric Skin and Wound Care.* Wounds UK Publishing, Aberdeen

Hester NKO (1979) The preoperational child's reaction to immunization. *Nurs Res* **28**: 250–4

Howard R (2003) Current status of pain management in children. *JAMA* **290**: 2464–9

Howard R, Carter B, Curry J et al (2008) *Good Practice in Post-Operative and Procedural Pain Management.* The Association of Paediatric Anaesthetists, Great Ormond Street Hospital for Children NHS Trust. Available online at: www.ich.ucl.ac.uk/clinical_information/clinical_guidelines/ext_guideline_00017/APA_Guideline_part_10.pdf

Hunt K, Peters J (2007) Guideline for sucrose administration for painful procedures. Pain control service CNS. Great Ormond Street Hospital for Children NHS Trust, London. Available online at: www.ich.ucl.ac.uk/

Johnson CC, Stevens BJ, Franck LS, Jack A, Stremler R, Platt R (1999) Factors explaining lack of response to heel-stick in pre-term newborns. *J Obstet Gynecol Neonatal Nurs* **28**: 587–94

Jonsdottir RB, Kristjansdottir G (2005) The sensitivity of the premature infant pain profile: PIPP to measure pain in hospitalised neonates. _J Eval Clinical Pract_ 11(6): 598–605

Laterjet J (2002) The management of pain associated with dressing changes in patients with burns. _World Wide Wounds_. Available online at: www.worldwidewounds.com/2002/november/Latarjet/Burn-Pain-At-Dressing-Changes.html [accessed 18 September 2008]

Mather C, Denyer J (2008) Removing dressings in epidermolysis bullosa. _Nurs Times_ 104(14): 46–8

Meaume S, Teot L, Lazareth I, Martini J, Bohbot S (2004) The importance of pain reduction through dressing selection in routine wound management: the MAPP study. _J Wound Care_ 13(10): 409–13

Molan PC (2001) Honey as a topical antibacterial agent for the treatment of infected wounds. _World Wide Wounds_. Available online at: www.worldwidewounds.com/2001/november/Molan/honey-as-topical-agent.html [accessed 18 September 2008]

Morash D, Fowler K (2004) An evidenced-based approach to changing practice: using sucrose for infant analgesia. _J Paediatr Nurs_ 19(5): 366–70

Morris C, Emsley P, Marland E, Meulenaere F, White RJ (2008) An observational study of dressings with soft silicone adhesive technology to manage the wounds of paediatric patients. _Paed Nurs_ in press

Rauch DA (1998) Use of ketamine in a pain management protocol for repetitive procedures. _Paediatrics_ 102(2 part 1): 404–5

St-Laurent-Gagnon T, Bernard-Bonnin AC, Villeneuve E (1999) Pain evaluation in preschool children and by their parents. _Acta Paediatr_ 88: 422–7

Stevens B, Yamada J, Ohlsson A (2004) Sucrose for analgesia in newborn infants undergoing painful procedures. Cochrane Database of Systematic Reviews 2004, Issue 2. Art. No: CD001069

Stinson J, Kavanagh T, yamada J, Gill N, Stevens B (2006) Systematic review of the psychometric properties, interpretability and feasibility of self-report pain intensity measures for use in clinical trials in children and adolescents. _Pain_ 125(1–2): 143–57

Syrjala KL, Abrams JR (1996) Hypnosis and imagery in the treatment of pain. In: Gatchel RJ, Turk D, eds. _Psychological Approaches to Pain Management: a Practitioner's Handbook_. Guilford Press, New York: 231–58

Uman LS, Chambers CT, McGrath PJ, Kisely S (2006) Psychological interventions for needle-related procedural pain and distress in children and adolescents. _Cochrane Database Syst Rev_ 4: CD005179

Watterson G, Denyer J (2006) Skin symptoms. In: Goldman A, Hain R, Liben S, eds. _Oxford Textbook of Palliative Care for Children_. Oxford University Press, New York: 454 (chap 28)

Watterson G, Howard R, Goldman A (2004) Peripheral opioids in inflammatory pain. *Arch Dis Childhood* **89**: 679–81

Whitaker B (2003) *The Effects of Distraction, Relaxation and Guided Imagery on Procedural Fear and Pain in Children*. University of Ballarat, Australia

White RJ (2005) Evidence for atraumatic soft silicone wound dressing use. *Wounds UK* **1**(3): 104–10

Wong D, Baker C (1988) Pain in children: comparison of assessment scales. *Pediatr Nurs* **14**(1): 9–17

Wound Academy, Mölnlycke Health Care (2004) *Issues in Paediatric Wound Care: Minimising Trauma and Pain*. Report from a Multidisciplinary Advisory Group. Mölnlycke Health Care, Göteborg, Sweden

Wound Academy, Mölnlycke Health Care (2005) *Issues in Neonatal Wound Care: Minimising Trauma and Pain*. Report from an Independent Advisory Group. Mölnlycke Health Care Wound Academy, Göteborg, Sweden

CHAPTER 6

WOUND PAIN IN PALLIATIVE CARE

Patricia Grocott and Emma Briggs

Palliative care comprises the study and management of patients with active, progressive and advanced disease for whom the prognosis is limited and the focus of care is on the quality of life (Doyle *et al*, 2004). Many aspects of palliative care are applicable to the care of patients with curative illness, including the diagnosis of pain and provision of pain relief.

Palliative wound care refers to the care of patients with wounds that are non-healing or hard to heal because the underlying cause of the wound cannot be eliminated, or the patient's condition militates against healing. Examples of the former are individuals whose cancer infiltrates the skin, and is resistant to treatment, and infants and young adults with epidermolysis bullosa; examples of the latter are frail, elderly people at the end of life with pressure ulcers.

The population of patients that falls into the palliative wound care group has not been defined in terms of population statistics. In addition, there are sensitivities around labelling patients 'palliative' when the term has connotations of end of life care, which may not be appropriate for a particular individual. There is, however, growing recognition, in the US in particular, of the importance of palliative wound care, not least because the number of patients that fall within this group are increasing, and the fact that they are heavily dependent on healthcare resources, including wound care products (Ennis, 2005). Epidemiological data from the US illustrates the proportion of a given patient population that may be affected, and also the dependency. For example, a cross-sectional study and retrospective records review of patients in a large urban/suburban US hospice by Tippett (2005) indicates that of 383 hospice patients, 35% had skin wounds, of which 50% were pressure ulcers. In a case series of 192 consecutive patients referred for wound consultation, the average age of patients was 82, 67% of patients were female, patients had numerous comorbidities, and 40% of all wounds were pressure ulcers. Ennis (2005) quotes a figure of 26–28% of wounds seen in US outpatient clinics as not healing. These authors conclude that the magnitude of the problem will increase as a result of changing demographics and an increased incidence of chronic disease, at enormous cost to both patients and service provision.

Patients most commonly identified within the palliative wound care group are those with fungating malignant disease and the frail elderly (McDonald and Lesage, 2005). Key recurring questions arise, however, as to when the goals of wound healing change to palliation, and whether interventions are actually different. It could be argued that palliative wound care is essentially good wound care practice, in conjunction with supportive care to the patient, their family and social group, and structured around three core principles:

- treatment and palliation of underlying causes
- local wound management
- symptom management.

The focus of this chapter is a key aspect of symptom management: wound pain. The knowledge base and expertise for managing wound pain are drawn from physiology, psychology, symptom management in cancer and palliative care, pharmacology, theory and frameworks to guide wound management and the role of dressing products. This knowledge and skill is then applied in what can be very challenging and highly individual clinical and patient circumstances. The pain experienced can be multi-dimensional and include sources of pain that are related to comorbid conditions, as well as the wound. Pain management and palliative wound care can be seen as advanced clinical practice, requiring sound knowledge and skills, dedicated care from a multiprofessional team, creativity, and accountability.

This chapter will illustrate the multifactorial aspects of pain in palliative wound care drawing on two examples of patients with advanced fungating breast disease, lymphoedema and brachial nerve plexopathy who participated in Grocott's study (2000). These case histories are used to illustrate how two patients with similar physical conditions responded in different ways to their very difficult circumstances, including approaches to relieving physical pain and emotional distress. Case A, for example, clearly experienced all-consuming suffering, which Dame Cicely Saunders described as 'total pain'. This concept indicates the intensity and extreme nature of what can be experienced by an individual as a result of the physical, psychological, social and spiritual impact of advanced disease (Saunders, 1964).

The chapter will outline three core principles of palliative wound care in relation to pain, highlighting different sources of pain experienced by patients with advanced disease. These complicate pain assessment and impact on the pain experienced during interventions, such as wound dressing changes and personal care. Given the total, multidimensional pain experienced by palliative care patients with wounds, a multi-modal approach is needed for assessment and management. Pharmacological and non-pharmacological methods are reviewed along with using drug combinations and the practice of prescribing licensed drugs for unlicensed purposes will be outlined.

Palliative wound care structured around three core principles

Principle 1: Treatment and palliation of the underlying disease or condition

As with any wound, the underlying cause needs to be diagnosed and treated if at all possible. If the cause is tumour infiltration of the skin leading to a fungating wound, conventional anti-cancer treatments may be effective. In addition, treatments such as radiotherapy can be used palliatively to relieve symptoms such as pain and local bleeding, and reduce tumour size (Pearson and Mortimer, 2004; Grocott, 2007). As is well established, if the cause of the wound is unrelieved pressure with friction and shearing leading to the loss of tissue viability and a pressure ulcer, these factors need to be eliminated if the wound is to heal (Grocott and Dealey, 2004).

Principle 2: Local wound management

Wound dressings in conjunction with symptom management can significantly relieve the physical and psychosocial problems, and therefore the overall impact of these wounds (Lawton, 2000; Lund-Nielsen _et al_, 2005). Local wound management is determined by the location, size and shape of the wounds, together with presenting problems such as exudate, odour, and maceration of the peri-wound skin. Local pain is related to specific interventions such as dressing changes. With modern wound dressings, cleansing solutions and careful dressing technique, dressing adherence and trauma at dressing changes should be unnecessary and avoidable sources of pain. That said, patients with long-term skin conditions and wounds, such as recessive dystrophic epidermolysis bullosa, can experience particular forms of pain (hyperalgesia and allodynia), which are difficult to manage during dressing changes (Abercrombie *et al*, 2008). In addition, there are no dedicated wound dressings for palliative care and the same products for mainstream wound care need to be adapted. When the wounds exceed the sizes of dressings, multiple overlapped dressings may need to be applied. When the dressings slip they can be further sources of pain, trauma and indignity that are not easily avoided. There is a real need for dressing designs to accommodate the scale and severity of wounds seen in palliative care.

Principle 3: Symptom management

Patients with advanced disease may experience a number of unpleasant and distressing symptoms. With regard to symptoms localised to the wound, these include: pain, soreness and irritation from excoriated skin conditions, odour, and bleeding. Pruritis (itch) is another unpleasant and poorly understood symptom, which is apparently mediated via pain pathways but it is not known why an individual will experience pruritis as opposed to pain. What is known is that it is a very difficult symptom to control, and for a number of patients pain is preferable to pruritis (Zycliz, 2004).

Symptoms may be interrelated, with more than one problem needing to be addressed at a given time. For example, a fungating wound may bleed easily, be malodorous and also painful. If the wound becomes infected the pain, odour and bleeding problems are exacerbated, and may include rapid extension of the wound (Vowden and Cooper, 2006). It is important therefore to diagnose the infection problem because accurate diagnosis and treatment can reduce the severity of the problems, including local wound pain.

As described in *Chapter 1*, when damaged skin has healed and returned to normal, the once sensitised nociceptive system should return to a pre-sensitised state, without pain. With advanced disease and wounds, patients can be in a permanent sensitised state and experience persistent pain, both nociceptive and neuropathic in nature. In these conditions, low intensity stimuli, such as a gentle stroke, can produce pain perception (allodynia), and a more intense stimulus, such as dressing removal, can produce an increased response to pain (hyperalgesia). Hyperalgesia can be experienced at the site of the damaged tissue but also in healthy tissue in another location. In addition to the evident multidimensional nature of pain that may be experienced in advanced disease, there are other complex aspects of human functioning at the emotional level which can affect pain, such as personality, life experiences, and social relationships (Breitbart *et al*, 2004).

Assessment of pain

A comprehensive pain assessment is fundamental to effective pain management and has to move beyond simply rating intensity level. Pain assessment with palliative care patients should reflect the multidimensional experience that pain is. Understanding the total pain and individual experiences helps to identify appropriate medication, non-drug approaches, and strategies for minimising the effects of pain and maximising independence and control. Successful pain assessment is achieved through effective communication with the patient and their family, providing time, setting pain management targets and documentation and evaluation (Briggs, 2005).

Effective communication within a trusting relationship is essential, as people may be reluctant to report pain to healthcare professionals, language may be a barrier or the terminology used to describe their symptoms may be different. Some prefer the term discomfort, aching or hurting, although using these phrases does not mean that pain is less intense or has less of an impact (Briggs, 2005). Sensitivity is required to obtain information from patients and family, especially as their disease progresses and assessment focuses more on non-verbal signs of pain and discomfort. A comprehensive assessment needs time and patience to allow the expression of the personal experience, and the use of pain scales recognises the potential for becoming tired easily and the need to pace the assessment process.

Sensitive questioning should explore pain location (which may not be confined to the wound site), underlying causes, intensity, quality, aggravating factors, timing, meaning and impact of the pain on the individual and existing pain management strategies. Assessment scales currently available do not contain all of these important elements and rigorous research is needed to test these tools in palliative care patients (Hølen *et al*, 2006). The pain assessment tools that have been developed measure key aspects such intensity and quality of the pain. These include numerical rating scales (0–5, 0–10), verbal rating scales (none, mild, moderate, or severe pain), visual analogue scale (10 cm line with 'no pain at one end and 'worst pain imaginable' at the other), and the short-form McGill Pain Questionnaire, to name but a few.

Choice of tool depends on the preference and cognitive ability of the individual, but it is important to identify a system of measuring and documenting intensity of pain. Assessing pain at rest, during movement and wound dressing changes is important and provides insight into the pattern of pain experienced. Regular use of scales also provides people with a language and terms to communicate their pain to healthcare professionals. Tools can also help to negotiate pain management goals which can relate to intensity (mild pain to maximum), or be activity related (to be comfortable enough to be able to dress independently). Finally, evaluation and documentation is essential and there are specific charts available (e.g. Bercovitch *et al*, 2002), but these are not always linked to treatment outcomes or goals. TELER is a generic system of clinical note-making with clinical indicators that offers this advantage (*Figure 6.1*). It focuses on measuring the relationship between patient treatment and care, and outcomes. The clinical indicator comprises an ordinal scale with six reference points, where 5 is the goal and 0 is the worst case scenario to be avoided or ameliorated. Core clinical knowledge and expertise in relation to symptom management and wound care are embedded

Code	
5	Pain controlled by the medicine
4	Aware of pain about 30 minutes before the next dose
3	For about an hour I was waiting for the next dose because of pain
2	Relief for about two hours after taking the medicine, then the pain returned
1	Some relief after taking the medicine, but it did not last long (less than one hour)
0	Pain not controlled by the medicine

Figure 6.1: TELER indicator: Wound pain due to underlying disease — effectiveness of four-hourly medications

to provide a focused rationale for interventions (Browne _et al_, 2004; Grocott _et al_, 2005).

Two types of indicators have been adopted for wound care: function and component indicators. The function indicators trace change in a given patient problem, from worst case (code 0) to achievement of the intended treatment goal (code 5). _Figure 6.2_ illustrates a function indicator for pain measurement, which is underpinned by the World Health Organization (WHO) recommendations, which are expanded on later in this chapter, that analgesics should be administered in a regular pattern to avoid patients experiencing pain. This indicator measures whether the patient experiences pain during a four-hourly regime, the detail of which will be charted on their drug chart. Component indicators capture the individual patient experience of a problem, illustrated in _Figure 6.2_, comprising five statements of a patient's experience of peri-wound soreness and local interventions.

Three forms of data are generated from the system: factual information about disease aetiology and treatment; written observations by clinicians; and numerical TELER codes, which include the patient's perspectives and experiences.

The psychological and emotional components of pain are emerging as being at least as important as the complex physiological processes that give rise to it. While pharmacological approaches remain the mainstay of pain management, increasingly, non-pharmacological approaches are being adopted and are acknowledged in this chapter.

Pharmacological approaches to palliative wound pain

The principles governing the use of three classes of analgesics (non-opioid, opioid, adjuvant) have been outlined in the WHO Method for the Relief of Cancer Pain (www.who.int/cancer/palliative/painladder/en/). Definitions of the drugs in each class are given in _Box 6.1_. The WHO principles of analgesic administration have been adopted in palliative care for patients with non-malignant conditions (Twycross and Wilcock, 2007). The WHO Pain Ladder (_Figure 6.3_) is a three-step process for pain relief (_Chapter 8_).

The WHO Pain Ladder is built on the premise that if pain occurs there should be prompt administration of analgesics: non-opioids for mild pain, followed, as necessary, with weak opioids then strong opioids, until the patient is free of pain. Adjuvant analgesics (e.g.

> **Please construct five statements with the patient, which define the scope of the problem. The statements here are examples of the sorts of issues patients have raised**
>
> a. Better when exposed to the air
> b. Worse when the dressings were wet
> c. Worse with heat
> d. Barrier film had dried out before she applied it, so no protection
> e. Of all the problems, this one could be avoided

Figure 6.2: TELER indicator: Peri-wound soreness from exudate — personal experiences

low dose tricyclic antidepressants or anticonvulsants) can be used at each stage to treat the neuropathic element of the pain. To maintain freedom from pain, the WHO recommends that patients take their drugs 'by the clock', rather than when they experience pain. This three-step approach of administering the right drug in the right dose, and related to individual patient episodes of pain, is considered to be an effective and cost-effective approach to pain relief.

Patients experience pain in well recognised patterns including:

- persistent background pain, where analgesia is inadequate
- breakthrough pain, where pain is experienced spontaneously in circumstances when it is usually well controlled by the prescribed analgesia
- end-of-dose failure pain, where a modified release preparation is prescribed and pain is experienced before the next dose should be administered
- incident pain, where pain is associated with specific movement or an intervention such as a dressing change.

Each of these manifestations of pain may indicate a clinical intervention in terms of systemic or topical analgesia. The WHO also indicates that in situations of persistent pain other interventions may be needed, such as surgical dissection of nerves. In palliative care, spinal analgesia may also be administered by an anaesthetist when more standard systemic analgesia does not give optimal outcomes (Twycross and Wilcock, 2007).

A key feature of pain and symptom management in palliative care is that up to a quarter of all prescriptions are written for licensed drugs given for unlicensed indications and/or via an unlicensed route. A chapter in the third edition of the *Palliative Care Formulary* sets out clearly the regulations and responsibilities in relation to prescribing outside the licence (Twycross and Wilcock, 2007: xviii–xxi).

Topical opioids are a key example of such practice in relation to wounds, which remains controversial until more research evidence is accrued. It is now established that nociceptive nerve fibres contain peripheral opioid receptors that are silent until local tissue is inflamed. Topical morphine and

> ### Box 6.1: Classes of analgesics
>
> **Non-opioid:** aspirin, paracetamol, non-steroidal anti-inflammatory drugs, e.g. ibuprofen
> **Weak opioid:** for mild to moderate pain, e.g. codeine
> **Opioid:** for moderate to severe pain, e.g. morphine/fentanyl, systemically, transdermally or topically
> **Adjuvant:** a drug that has a primary indication other than pain but can relieve painful conditions, e.g. antidepressants, anticonvulsants, muscle relaxants, local anaesthetics, transcutaneous electrical nerve stimulation (TENS), acupuncture, relaxation techniques

diamorphine have been used successfully to relieve otherwise unrelieved pain from local ulcers (Back and Finlay, 1995; Krajnik and Zycliz, 1997; Grocott, 2000). At present, there are no 'off-the-shelf' preparations and topical opioids are made for individual patients. Further information can be found in the *Palliative Care Formulary*, and practitioners need to refer to local prescribing policies and procedures (Twycross and Wilcock, 2007: 279).

Non-pharmacological approaches to palliative wound pain

These approaches to palliating wound pain can be divided into physical and non-physical interventions. Non-pharmacological approaches draw on the creative skills of individual clinicians, patients and their families ensuring a multimodal approach to pain management. Techniques can promote relaxation, stimulate the body's own natural opioids (endorphins, dynorphins and enkephalins) promote autonomy, boost self-esteem and a sense of well-being. Non-drug approaches can address the total pain an individual may experience, as illustrated in Case history B.

Physical interventions include massage, repositioning, acupuncture, and transcutaneous electrical nerve stimulation (TENS) (*Table 6.1; Chapter 9*). Some of these require additional recognised training and qualifications and clinicians are accountable for their use. Careful patient assessment, evaluation and documentation of the outcomes are needed.

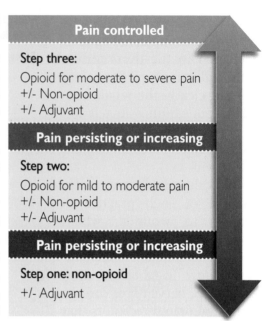

Psychosocial interventions include relaxation techniques, aromatherapy, guided imagery, support groups, family counselling, education, biofeedback, and psychotherapy. In addition, hospices such as St Christopher's Hospice, London have a Creative Living Centre (www.stchristophers.org.uk/page.cfm/link=48), where physical care needs are looked after in conjunction with social, emotional and creative needs.

Figure 6.3: The steps of the WHO Pain Ladder

Distraction techniques and guided imagery can be particularly useful as an adjuvant to analgesics for procedural pain, such as at wound dressing changes. Guided imagery has been found to be useful for people with cancer pain (Kwekkeboom *et al*, 2003) and can adjust the meaning of pain for people with regular use (Lewandowski *et al*, 2005). A simple example of the technique is provided in *Box 6.2*.

The care of patients with painful wounds and advanced disease can be daunting. The following case histories illustrate the challenges presented and the ways in which clinicians have deployed pharmacological and non-pharmacological approaches to pain relief and comfort.

Case history A

Ms A was a 48-year-old woman with extensive localised chest wall disease from a primary breast cancer (*Figure 6.4*). The 'wound' extended into the dermis of the chest wall with separate wounds on her left arm, which was lymphoedematous. The damaged skin was very sensitive.

Table 6.1: Common complementary and alternative therapies for pain management (based on Wigens, 2006)

Therapy	Description
Acupuncture	Traditional Chinese therapy involving the insertion of fine needles into specific points on the skin related to meridians, lines of energy. Seems to work by promoting the production of natural opioids and diverting or changing painful sensations that are sent to the brain
Aromatherapy and massage	Massage involves manual, rhythmic movement of soft tissues and muscles to reduce anxiety, stress, muscular tension and fatigue. Aromatherapy oils are plant oils that are reported to have a number of properties and are massaged into the skin or inhaled
Hypnotherapy	Hypnotherapy helps a person reach a deep, trance-like state to induce relaxation and use of the unconscious mind
Homeopathy	Based on the idea that 'like can be cured with like', homeopathy uses diluted, low-dose preparations to induce similar symptoms
Guided imagery	Used to promote relaxation by directing thoughts and images. Particularly useful for procedural pain such as at wound dressing changes
Reflexology	Varying pressure is applied to the reflex areas of the feet or hands based on the idea that every part of the body is connected, and pathways terminate in the hands and feet
Relaxation	Techniques used to induce progressive muscle relaxation and can include music, biofeedback (learning to use relaxation to achieve an end point) and distraction
Shiatsu	Practitioner's body is used to apply pressure to various parts of the patient's body in combination with stretches, joint rotations and manipulation
Transelectrical nerve stimulation (TENS)	An electronic device that produces a small electrical current through electrodes placed on the skin. Particularly useful for neuropathic pain

Her symptoms comprised soreness and itching, around the nipple region in particular. Water was soothing, for example, during a shower or Jacuzzi bath, but after a period of exposure to water, it had the reverse effect because of nipple contraction. She was exquisitely sensitive to saline, expressed here in her own words: '... I hit the roof'.

Box 6.2: An example of guided imagery technique

1. Sit in a comfortable position where you feel relaxed.

2. Close your eyes and focus on your breathing, slowing down your breathing and imagine breathing out the stress and anxiety you feel.

3. When you are feeling relaxed, imagine yourself in a place where you feel calm, warm, safe and secure. This could be on holiday, on a beach or simply at home in your own bed.

4. Think about what you can see, feel, hear and test to make your visualisation as real as possible. Spend as much time as you can exploring your place.

5. When you are ready, become aware of your slow regular breathing again for a minute and then count backwards from ten and open your eyes.

Symptoms related to a comorbid condition

Her left arm was lymphodematous, grossly swollen and with brachial nerve plexopathy, which is usually attributed to damage to the nerves after surgical excision of axillary lymph nodes and/or radiotherapy to the axilla. The condition was managed with lympoedema bandaging although staff were not convinced it was reducing the swelling, but the treatment was preventing it from progressing. The application of the bandages aggravated the cutaneous soreness and itch problems. The dressing changes aggravated the acute pain in her arm and neck from the brachial nerve plexopathy. This was evident when she had to sit up for the dressing change, and hold her heavy arm in order that the dressings and a retention garment could be applied.

Wound dressing problems

The dressings were too small to cover the extensive broken areas on the chest wall, requiring several overlapping dressings. At this point a non-adherent silicone mesh dressing was being applied with gamgee roll and a front-fastening, elasticated lumbar/abdominal support garment to hold the dressings in place. The silicone mesh dressings were inherently unstable because they could not be fitted on to areas

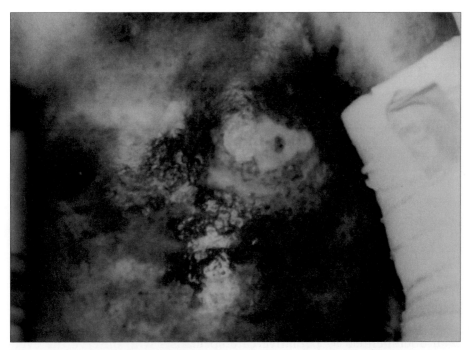

Figure 6.4: Extensive fungating tumour from primary breast cancer symptoms local to damaged skin

of intact skin, as recommended by the manufacturers. The dressings moved around, frequently ending up in a rolled ball, which exacerbated the soreness and itch problems, together with the heat generated by the dressing layers. Dressing changes were required at least three times daily, and these were lengthy and required additional medication. In her words: '... I am fed up being mucked about'.

Emotional pain

This woman appeared to embody the concept of 'total pain' alluded to in the introduction to this chapter, which was understandable given the nature of her advanced disease. This extract from the research field notes illustrates how her emotional pain manifested:

> ... The nurse said the only way she could describe what happened last week was that 'she lost it'. Midazolam (benzodiazepine — a short-acting sedative) did not touch her; she needed methotrimeprazine (a sedative drug with antipsychotic,

tranquillising, anxiolytic, and analgesic properties). She was inconsolable. The doors were open to the ward studio where there is a full-length mirror. She caught sight of herself and dropped to her knees in total despair.

Pharmacological interventions

Pain medication followed step three of the WHO Pain Ladder and included drugs for nociceptive pain, including two non-opioid drugs (paracetamol and a non-steroidal anti-inflammatory drug), a strong opioid (oral morphine), and an adjuvant drug for neuropathic pain (a tricyclic antidepressant, amitriptyline). At dressing changes a dose of oramorphine was given before, during and after the dressing change (Twycross and Wilcock, 2007). As her disease progressed, her pain and emotional distress were not relieved and she required increased frequency and dosage of analgesic and anti-anxiolytic drugs. This pattern of increased use of pharmacological interventions has been well documented by palliative care specialists who observe the ever-increasing frequency and dosage of drugs when patients experience unrelieved suffering (Dunlop, 1998).

Non-pharmacological interventions

These were focused on reducing the impact of the dressing changes. The nurses said they had tried to engage this patient in relaxation techniques, as they predicted 'the going was bound to be tough', but she could not get on with this approach.

Three nurses assisted with dressing changes, with one nurse dedicated to supporting her back and arm. Several pauses were factored into the procedure to allow her to rest back on the pillows to relieve the pain in her arm and neck. Her lymphoedema bandaging and the arm dressing were done at a different time once she had recovered from the dressing change, which followed her personal care.

The dressing protocol was reviewed and the silicone mesh dressings were substituted with large occlusive gel sheets (40x40 cms to front of chest; 15x20 cms to her arm) and the lumbar support garment to hold the chest wall sheets in place. The patient apparently described the gel sheet as 'a blessing'. The nurses said that while she was asleep they changed the dressing on the front of the chest. The soreness and irritation were relieved by the occlusive gel sheet and, together with the 'corset', simplified the dressing system and thereby reduced the trauma and pain of the dressing changes. Added benefits of the dressing were debridement of dry crusts on the chest wall, which if knocked bled profusely (*Figures* 6.5 and 6.6). Given the all-consuming nature of her pain experience, it was remarkable that she was able to

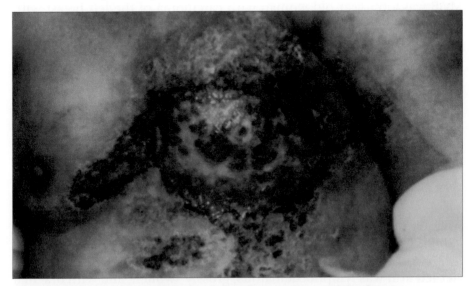

Figure 6.5: Extensive fungation of the chest wall: pre-debridement

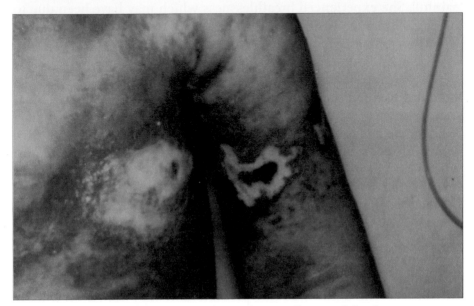

Figure 6.6: Extensive fungation of the chest wall: post-debridement

discriminate between a successful local intervention to the wounds and the rest of her situation.

Case history B

Ms B was a 65-year-old woman with carcinoma of the left breast with advanced local spread in anterior and posterior chest wall, shoulder and axilla (*Figures 6.7* and *6.8*). She was originally diagnosed after a routine mammogram.

Symptoms local to damaged skin

She experienced soreness and discomfort when dressings were removed. She also experienced soreness and bleeding when showering. She was very clear that the word 'pain' was not appropriate to her situation.

Symptoms related to a comorbid condition

Her left arm was lymphoedematous, grossly swollen, and with brachial nerve plexopathy, it was heavy and she expressed these symptoms as 'painful'. She experienced breathlessness which may have been due to the circumferential oedema of the chest wall, which limited her chest expansion. She also experienced facial swelling.

Wound dressing problems

Exudate management and fitting dressings to cover the extensive broken areas on her chest wall, arm and axilla were major problems. When the chest wall was exposed the exudate was not obvious. However, as soon as hydrophilic, absorbent materials were applied (alginate, semi-occlusive foams) they soaked through requiring several dressing changes in a day. On removal, the dressings 'tugged'.

She was unable to lift her arm because of a loss of movement associated with the brachial nerve plexopathy; cleaning and fitting dressings to the axilla was not possible and they relied on a daily shower to maintain a degree of hygiene.

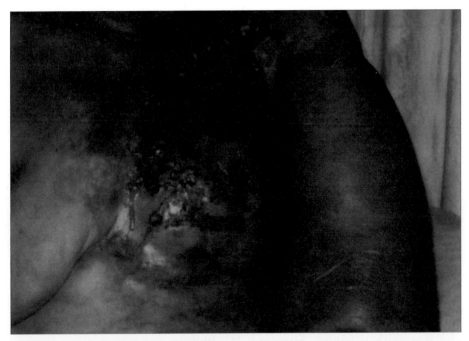

Figure 6.7: Advanced tumour infiltration of the chest wall: anterior view

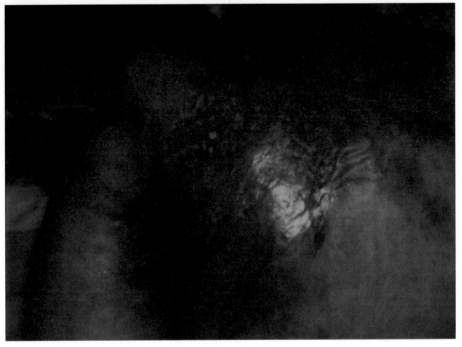

Figure 6.8: Advanced tumour infiltration of the chest wall: posterior view

Dressing changes lasted anything from one to one and a half hours, after which she was exhausted. Her lymphoedema bandaging was done separately by the physiotherapist once she had recovered from the dressing change.

Emotional pain

She said the wound had become the focus of daily life. She described the 'ordeal' of the dressings, which she said she coped with by 'taking a walk'. She explained that she had had rheumatic fever as a child, and had been in bed for most of a year. The pain was very bad and the consultant told her that she had to 'take a walk in the woods'. She said she had a constant sense of having to face what had gone before and felt that if we could simplify the dressing regime, it would be less of an ordeal.

In relation to the dressings and uncontrolled exudate, she explained that if the dressing gives, it poured into her lap. This happened when she was with a friend. She said: '… luckily she was a close friend'. She also said she enjoyed going to Fine Arts Society lectures, but she suddenly feels the dressing going and says to herself, 'oh no' and quickly removes herself. She described the soiling, especially the bedclothes. She said the washing is everywhere, 'you can never get away from it [the wound]'.

She talked about the difference between coping with dressings at home and being 'indulged and pampered' in the hospice. She said she was just sitting back and accepting the luxury. She was clearly worried about managing at home. In the event, her condition suddenly deteriorated and she died in the hospice.

Pharmacological interventions

As for case history A, the pain medication followed step three of the WHO Pain Ladder and included drugs for nociceptive pain including one non-opioid drug (a non-steroidal anti-inflammatory drug), a strong opioid, which was initially administered as a twelve-hourly, slow-release preparation and changed to a four-hourly regime when she experienced breakthrough pain (oral morphine solution), and an adjuvant drug for neuropathic pain (a tricyclic antidepressant, amitriptyline) (Twycross and Wilcock, 2007).

Non-pharmacological interventions

These comprised a combination of the visualisation techniques she adopted herself, and local wound interventions aimed at simplifying the wound care protocol, reducing the frequency of dressing changes and the leakage. Apart from the use of a barrier cream to reduce the tug of the dressings on removal, the local wound interventions were not successful in bringing the exudate under control or reducing the burden of the interventions.

Conclusions

This chapter has outlined three core principles of palliative wound care and has focused on wound pain and the care of patients with advanced disease. The knowledge base is principally drawn from symptom management in cancer and palliative care and pharmacology, and also wound care. Wound pain in palliative care can be complex, it is a highly individual experience and multi-dimensional embracing the total pain that Dame Cicely Saunders described. This complexity means that pain assessment, management and palliative wound care are clearly located in advanced clinical practice. The hallmarks of such practice are knowledgeable and dedicated practitioners working within a multiprofessional team who can also be creative, and demonstrate their accountability through sensitive patient assessment and outcome measurement.

References

Abercombie EM, Mather CA, Hon J, Graham-King P and Pilllay E (2008) Recessive dystrophic epidermolysis bullosa. Part 2. Care of the adult patient. _Br J Nurs_ 17(6): S6–10

Back IN, Finlay I (1995) Analgesic effect of topical opioids on painful skin ulcers. _J Pain Symptom Control_ 10(7): 493

Breitbart W, Payne D, Passik SD (2004) Psychological and psychiatric interventions in pain control. In: Doyle D, Hanks G, Cherny NI, Calman K, eds. _Oxford Textbook of Palliative Medicine._ 3rd edn. Oxford University Press, Oxford: 424–38

Bercovitch M, Waller A, Adunsky A (2002) Multidimensional continuous assessment chart (MCPAC) for terminal cancer patients: a preliminary report. *Am J Hospice Palliative Care* 19(6): 419–25

Briggs E (2005) Pain. In: Heath H, Watson R, eds. *Older People: Assessment for Health and Social Care*. Age Concern, London

Browne N, Grocott P, Cowley S, *et al* (2004) Woundcare Research for Appropriate Products (WRAP): Validation of the TELER Method Involving Users. *Int J Nurs Stud* 41: 559–71

Doyle D, Hanks G, Cherny NI, Calman K (2004) Introduction. In: Doyle D, Hanks G, Cherny NI, Calman K, eds. *Oxford Textbook of Palliative Medicine*. 3rd edn. Oxford University Press, Oxford: 1

Dunlop R (1998) *Cancer: Palliative Care*. Springer, London

Ennis W J, Vargas M, Lee C, Meneses P (2005) Palliative care and wound care: 2 emerging fields with similar needs for outcomes data. *Wounds: a compendium of clinical research and practice* 17(4): 99–104

Grocott P (2000) Palliative management of fungating malignant wounds. *J Community Nurs* 14(3): 31–40

Grocott P, Browne N, Richardson A (2003) Palliative Wound Care: optimising the use of classification systems. *Polish Palliative Med* 2(4): 222–32

Grocott P, Dealey C (2004) Skin problems in palliative care, nursing aspects. In: Doyle D, Hanks G, Cherny N, Calman K, eds. *Oxford Textbook of Palliative Medicine*. 3rd edn. Oxford Medical Publications, Oxford: 629–40

Grocott P, Browne N, Cowley S (2005) WRAP: Defining clinical needs for fluid handling devices. *Wounds UK* 1(2): 11–18

Grocott P (2007) Care of patients with fungating malignant wounds. *Nurs Standard* 21(24): 57–66

Hølen JC, Polit C, Hjermstad MJ, *et al* (2006) Pain assessment tools: Is the content appropriate for use in palliative care? *J Pain Symptom Management* 32(6): 567–80

Johnson M (2006) Physiology of pain. In: White R, Harding K, eds. *Trauma and Pain in Wound Care*. Wounds UK, Aberdeen: 17–58

Krajnik M, Zylicz Z (1997) Topical morphine for cutaneous cancer pain. *Palliative Med* 11(4): 326

Kwekkeboom KL, Kneip J, Pearson L (2003) A pilot study to predict success with guided imagery for cancer pain. *Pain Management Nurs* 4(3): 112–23

Lawton J (2000) *The Dying Process: Patients' experiences of palliative care*. Routledge, London.

Lewandoswsli W, Good M, Drauker C (2005) Changes in the meaning of pain with the use of guided imagery. *Pain Management Nurs* 6(2): 58–67

Lund-Nielsen B, Muller K, Adamsen L (2005) Qualitative and quantitative evaluation of a new regimen for malignant wounds in women with advanced breast cancer. _J Wound Care_ **14**(2): 69–73

McDonald A, Lesage P (2006) Palliative management of pressure ulcers and malignant wounds in patients with advanced illness. _J Palliative Med_ **9**(1): 285–95

Pearson IC, Mortimer P (2004) Skin problems in palliative medicine: medical aspects. In: Doyle D, Hanks G, Cherny NI, Calman K, eds. _Oxford Textbook of Palliative Medicine_. 3rd edn. Oxford University Press, Oxford: 618–28

Saunders C (1964) The symptomatic treatment of incurable disease. _Prescribers J_ **4**(4): 68–73

Tippett A (2005) Wounds at the end of life. _Wounds_ **17**(4): 91–8

Twycross R, Wilcock A (2007) _Palliative Care Formulary PCF3_. Palliative Drugs.com Ltd. Nottingham University Hospitals NHS Trust, Nottingham. Available online at: www.palliativedrugs.com

Vowden P, Cooper R (2006) An integrated approach to managing wound infection. In: EWMA Position Document. _Management of wound infection_. London, MEP Ltd: 2–6

Wigens L (2006) The role of complementary and alternative therapies in pain management. In: MacLellan K, ed. _Management of Pain: A Practical Approach for Healthcare Professionals_. Nelson-Thorne, Cheltenham

World Health Organiszation (WHO) Pain Ladder. WHO, Geneva. Available online at: www.who.int/cancer/palliative/painladder/en/ [last accessed 18 August, 2008]

Zylicz Z (2004) An introduction to pruritis. In: Twycross R, Jones EA, eds. _Pruritus in Advanced Disease_. Oxford University Press, Oxford: 1–9

CHAPTER 7

MANAGING THE PAIN OF BURN WOUNDS

Keith Judkins and Laura Clark

A significant burn is one of the most painful injuries a person can suffer. Unfortunately, burn pain is also one of the most difficult to alleviate, as both its severity and duration are highly variable. Essential treatments, such as wound debridement, skin grafting and physiotherapy, can cause more pain initially but may diminish the pain experience overall. However, if direct pain is not well controlled, not only will the patient suffer immediately, but he or she may take longer to recover and may develop chronic pain. Worryingly, studies show that pain is frequently under-estimated and under-treated, even in specialist burn centres (Patterson *et al*, 2004).

In the short term, poorly managed pain may exacerbate burn hypermetabolism in major burns, contributing to under-nutrition, immunological impairment and sensitivity to infection. Long-term, prolonged pain will increase the risk of developing depression or post-traumatic stress disorder and by this and other mechanisms hinder recovery (Taal and Faber, 1997). Anxiety or depression may themselves heighten a patient's perception of pain, an unhappy vicious cycle that is difficult to break once established. Minor burn wounds, while easier to manage, are not immune from the long-term sequelae of badly controlled pain.

The majority of the population will suffer a minor burn at some point in their lives — ask any audience of lay people. These are trivial injuries which from the pain perspective can be treated as any other small wound, with simple analgesia, but other wound care caveats should be considered, particularly the time to heal and the importance of change in wound appearance and/or pain intensity, as signs of problems such as infection. Around 13,000 people require admission to hospital for burns every year in the United Kingdom, and of these, on average about 300 will die (British Burn Association, 2001).

Burn pain management is a vast and fascinating topic and this chapter must therefore focus on managing pain during burn dressings' procedures; however, to do so in isolation from the general management of the burn wound and its pain would skate unhelpfully over the many factors that influence procedural pain and make chronic pain more likely. The pathophysiology of wound pain is well described in *Chapter 1*; this chapter takes that complex understanding for granted, focuses on analgesia during burn wound management, has a little to say about children, and includes comment about the use of more drastic measures such as general anaesthesia.

Burn classification

Most burn wounds are caused by thermal injury, such as flame and scalds (generally hot water, sometimes other hot fluids, notably oil or fat) or by cold injury (frost-bite). Burn wounds as a result of electricity, chemicals, contact with hot structures and radiation are more rare (Hettiaratchy and Dziewulski, 2004). Classifying the burn by area and depth can be an indicator for the intensity of pain that might be anticipated, although some studies have not found this to be an accurate predictor (Perry and Heidrich, 1982; Atchison *et al*, 1991). It has been reported that burn pain intensity may vary with, but cannot be predicted by, factors such as age or sex (Latarjet and Choinière, 1995).

The burn area (the percent of total body surface area, or %tbsa) is most accurately classified using the Lund and Browder chart (*Figure 7.1*) (Wachtel *et al*, 2000). Smaller injuries can be assessed by comparison to the palmar surface of the patient's (not the assessor's) hand, which equates to somewhat less than 1%tbsa; this works for burns less than 5%tbsa, but can be dangerously inaccurate for larger burns (Hettiaratchy and Papini, 2004).

The depth of a burn is classified by description according to the extent of damage to the skin's layers (*Figure 7.2*). The terms 'first, second and third degree' for superficial, partial- and full-thickness burns are no longer used in the UK, although they are still to be found in many first aid manuals.

- *Superficial burns*, such as sunburn, damage only the epidermis and, as the nerves are intact, may be exquisitely painful especially during dressing changes.
- *Partial-thickness burns* are often referred to as 'dermal burns'

because the injury extends into, but not beyond, the dermis. They are usually subdivided according to the depth of tissue damage into superficial and deep dermal burns. Nerve endings are destroyed in the burned tissue but stimulated in deeper dermis layers, so significant pain can be anticipated.

- **Full-thickness burns** extend through all the skin's layers and may also affect the subcutaneous tissue, muscle or bone. Due to the

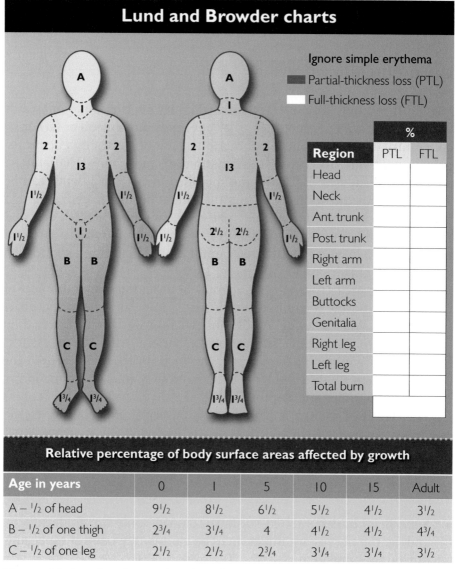

Figure 7.1: Lund and Browder chart for classifying total burn surface area

destruction of the nerve endings these burns are initially painless until the nerves start to regenerate. Nevertheless, inflammatory processes quickly stimulate pain in the immediate surroundings.

Nevertheless, it is futile to anticipate the pain experience from wound depth alone because the complex causation of wound pain means that no burn wound will remain pain-free for long (Choinière, 2003).

Most patients are likely to have more than one depth of burn, depending on the cause and pattern of injury. For example, a patient with a full-thickness burn, and therefore initially largely painless, may still be in pain from the surrounding partial-thickness burn. The inflammatory response will also spread to the surrounding unburned tissue causing hyperalgesia. Additionally, the greater the severity of a burn, the longer it will take to heal, with a greater requirement for treatment and interventions. It could therefore be anticipated that such a patient would perhaps suffer more, with more complex pain over time than someone with an initially more painful, but more quickly healing, superficial burn.

The healing process itself can cause pain. Full-thickness and most deep dermal burns require skin grafts. Prior to the graft, all necrotic tissue must be excised and this can cause further damage to regenerating nerve endings. Furthermore, at the donor skin site a new wound is generated, which is akin to a shallow dermal wound

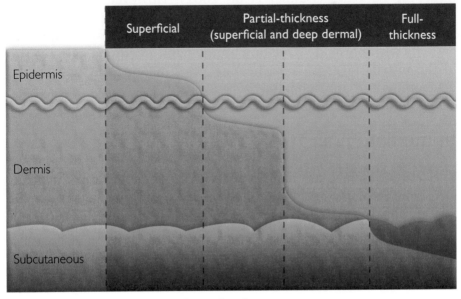

Figure 7.2: Diagram showing burn depths

with many cut nerve endings. The donor site may be more painful than the original burn wound. Nerve regeneration can be painful, and may have neuropathic elements such as tingling and itching. The prolonged and repetitive nature of burn wound pain, particularly in deeper wounds, is the reason why a significant proportion of patients go on to develop chronic abnormal sensation syndromes, including post-healing pain and intense itching (Dauber *et al*, 2002; Brooks *et al*, 2008).

Types of burn pain

The literature tends to differentiate burn pain into four groups (Patterson, 2004):

- immediate pain
- resting or background pain
- breakthrough pain
- procedural pain.

Chronic pain and paraesthesia, due to changes in the repaired nerve fibres, may also occur. One US study of 358 burns survivors found that 52% reported chronic pain, with a mean time since injury of 12 years (Dauber *et al*, 2002). However, as this was a postal questionnaire, it is possible that those who were still in pain were more likely to respond. Nevertheless, a significant number of patients with burns do develop chronic pain. Adequate pain control in the initial stages of burn healing can limit or even prevent the development of chronic pain.

Immediate pain

The level of immediate pain experienced following a burn depends on a variety of factors, including the depth and area of burn. The relationship is not linear but is influenced by the psyche and prior experiences of the patient, as well as the nature of the wound. Good initial management, such as cooling the burn as a first aid measure and providing prompt analgesia is essential, especially to minimise the pain inevitably caused by clinical staff when assessing the burn (Dearden *et al*, 2001).

Managing immediate pain

Intravenous analgesia using opiates is the modality of choice for larger burns, but may sometimes be necessary in minor injuries to gain initial pain control. Oral or intramuscular absorption may be unpredictable in large injuries (>5%tbsa), where fluid shifts cause temporary circulation deficits in muscle and gut tissues. Therefore, the administration of small incremental doses of opiates until control is achieved should be matched by vigilant attention to side-effects, such as respiratory depression and drowsiness, together with scrupulous knowledge of the pharmacokinetics of the drug used; the goal is comfort, not absence of pain. Oral or intravenous paracetamol may reduce the amount of opiate required.

Resting or background pain

Resting or background pain is the constant pain present at the site of injured tissue, and will include pain in the donor areas where skin has been harvested for grafts (Choinière, 2003). Background pain can vary from day to day, ranging in intensity from mild to severe and can often persist for weeks without any decrease over time. The treatment of background pain can be difficult without causing unpleasant side-effects such as nausea and itching. These factors, along with a fear of opioid dependency, may lead to insufficient analgesia being provided. David Patterson, a clinical psychologist with many years' experience in the management of pain in burn patients, states that there is 'no evidence that opioid addiction occurs more commonly in burns patients than in other populations requiring opioids for acute pain' (Patterson *et al*, 2004).

As the patient's experience of background burn pain has different components and varies both over time and between patients, pain management must be well evaluated and tailored to the individual (Latarjet and Choinière, 1995). These authors also stress that, 'pain sensitivity may increase over time, and all the more so if pain management has been inappropriate'. McCaffery and Pasero (1999) recommend that when patients are hospitalised, pain ratings for each type of pain should be recorded throughout the day to facilitate pain management, with the derived scores being used to influence the subsequent dosing regimen. A perception persists even in specialised burns units, that this is time-consuming and may not be feasible on a busy ward. However, Jonsson *et al* (1998) have shown that in practice diligent monitoring of pain intensity is not only feasible, but brings benefits in terms of patient satisfaction and recovery. A simple, four-point pain score regularly recorded and acted on is better than nothing in this respect.

Managing background pain

Background pain management is best addressed by a structured approach, such as that of the World Health Organization (WHO) analgesic ladder (*Figure 7.3*), developed for cancer pain but which has proved useful as a guide for managing many types of pain of varying intensity persistent over weeks or months. Pre-emptive, regular dosing supplemented by additional prescriptions for breakthrough pain is most effective in practice, provided the patient has freedom to refuse analgesia when completely pain-free. Patterson *et al* (2004) commented that when patients required hospitalisation, their burns will usually be severe enough to require opioids for effective analgesia. In lesser injuries, non-steroidal anti-inflammatory drugs (NSAIDs) and paracetamol (acetaminophen) can be remarkably effective when taken regularly, by reason of their anti-inflammatory, anti-prostaglandin actions (Pal *et al*, 1997). They also have an important role as adjuncts in all patients, as they can be opioid-sparing.

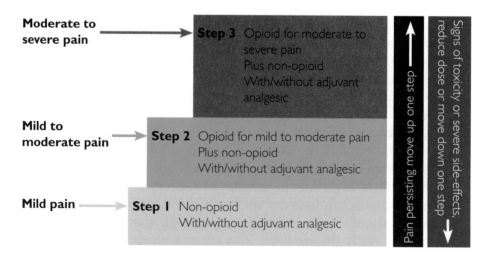

Figure 7.3: The WHO analgesic ladder (WHO, 2008)

NSAIDs should be used with caution in the elderly, those with moderate-to-severe asthma and those with renal impairment. Furthermore, due to the antiplatelet properties of NSAIDs and aspirin, patients with extensive open wounds or skin grafts may be at an increased risk of bleeding, especially during and immediately after skin grafting. Both paracetamol and NSAIDs can be made more effective by judicious, regular low doses of oral morphine, and the amount required provides a further indication of the adequacy of regular analgesia.

Synthetic opioid agents, such as tramadol, can be useful in the management of burns pain, especially when NSAIDs are contraindicated, but their effect can be disappointing. Other supplements such as clonidine or gabapentin may bring benefit if the opiate dose is high but partially effective, or if dose escalation is seen. Gabapentin has been proven to be effective in neuropathic pain (Melzack and Wall, 2003), counteracting spinal cord 'wind-up' (*Chapter 4*). Those who advocate its use in burn pain management hypothesise that there is a neuropathic element in immediate post-acute, as well as chronic burn pain. Cuignet *et al* (2007) reported that the adjunctive daily use of 2400 mg gabapentin in divided doses in addition to opioids, reduced both the pain score and morphine requirements of the patient and, therefore, reduced side-effects such as sedation, nausea and vomiting. They suggested that this was due to the ability of gabapentin to prevent central hyperalgesia induced by the burns. However, they acknowledge the small sample size ($n = 10$) and recommend further randomised studies. Finally, in this context of adjuncts to opioids, ketamine given orally may inhibit the expression of secondary hyperalgesia (Mikkelsen *et al*, 2000), although this has yet to be confirmed in the burns clinical setting.

Finally, it is important to remember that correct management of background and breakthrough pain can make a substantial positive difference to successful control of wound procedural pain; conversely, inadequate background pain control may increase patient anxiety about added pain during procedures, and thereby increase negative responses to necessary wound care interventions. This applies to minor wounds treated on an outpatient basis, as well as to inpatient treatment. Therefore, in dressings clinics, the patient's background pain experience at home should be specifically enquired about and stoic responses, e.g. 'I grin and bear it', 'I'm OK doc, really', 'It's worse at night, but I cope', should be probed. Reluctance to take painkillers at home should be counselled, particularly in respect of night pain (arguably the most psychologically demoralising part of the pain experience).

Non-pharmacological approaches to background pain have been investigated and found helpful in some instances. Burns have a major psychological impact on the patient, not only from the trauma of sustaining the injury and continual pain, but also from the disfigurement of the wound itself. Adjustment disorder, post-traumatic stress disorder, sleep disturbance, anxiety or depression may develop, hindering the patient's recovery and actually increasing their pain (Patterson *et al*, 1993; Franulic *et al*, 1996). Many burns centres employ psychologists or psychotherapists to help patients cope and adjust; it is no coincidence that these professionals also contribute significantly to pain control, as evidenced by their contributions to the burn pain literature (e.g. Patterson *et al*, 2004; Choinière, 2003).

Breakthrough pain

It is often difficult to distinguish between changes in background pain and additional pain caused by movement — both of which would be regarded as 'breakthrough pain'. For this reason, breakthrough pain has been dealt with alongside background pain (see above). Essentially, the same strategies apply for managing breakthrough pain as for background pain. It is vital to think of it, and to ensure breakthrough analgesia is included in the regimen (an 'as required' prescription of oral morphine three-hourly, for example). Excessive use of breakthrough analgesia is one factor that should normally trigger a review of the regular analgesia prescription.

Procedural pain

Procedural pain is experienced when therapies such as wound cleaning, debridement, dressing changes or physiotherapy are carried out. The debridement, cleansing and re-dressing of wounds stimulates the already hyperalgesic regenerating nerve endings and may cause intense pain. In addition, these procedures may need to be repeated several times a day for weeks or months. The inadequate control of pain prior to wound dressing changes could result in the anticipation of pain, thereby increasing patient anxiety and suffering. The requirement for anxiolytics such as benzodiazepines may then also increase. Byers *et al* (2001) showed that procedural pain was always much greater than resting pain, but the level of anxiety was not significantly different between the two. In contrast with resting pain, procedural pain matched the patients' estimation of what was an acceptable maximum level on average. Unsurprisingly, patients' anxiety about pain roughly correlated with the size of the wound, and the use of opiates and anxiolytics during a particular procedure correlated strongly with the patient's prior experience — more pain last time, more demand for pharmaceuticals this time (Byers *et al*, 2001).

Can the level of pain anxiety be predicted? According to Aaron *et al* (2001), it can. These authors have devised and evaluated a tool, the Burn-specific Pain Anxiety Score (BSPAS), which they say is the best predictor of procedural pain levels. While it does not predict resting pain levels, it is the only significant predictor of decreased physical functional after discharge. This study was undertaken in a specialised burn unit so the relevance of this tool to non-major burns is unclear, but it would not be unreasonable to suppose that good quality pain control is both humane and beneficial to overall recovery in all patients.

After the wound has been re-dressed, there is usually little or no residual pain additional to the background pain levels already being experienced. Indeed, for a while, background pain may be lessened after dressing changes. Much depends on the dressing being used. The use of wound dressings designed for maximum healing may also result in pain reduction (Barret *et al*, 2000).

Physiotherapy improves mobilisation and helps prevent scarring and contractures. In the early stages of wound healing, range of motion exercises may be best carried out when the patient is under general anaesthesia or sedated for wound debridement or dressing changes. Inadequate pain control at these times could mean the patient is later reluctant to mobilise, so hindering recovery. However, once active rehabilitation starts sedation must be relaxed so that the patient can be involved. Fortunately, by this stage, motivation to return to active independent living can mitigate pain unless earlier experiences have induced fear.

Managing procedural pain

Optimal treatment of the burn wound

The most important factor in achieving pain control during successive procedures for the burn wound is not, paradoxically perhaps, the analgesia component, but how the burn wound itself is managed. If not managed actively and appropriately (for more detail on appropriate management of burn wounds, see Papini, 2004), the wound has more potential to become chronic, pain relief will be harder to achieve, scarring will be worse and harder to manage, and chronic pain syndromes are more likely. There is no reason to believe that this is less true for small burns than it undoubtedly is for larger injuries, especially if the burn is in important areas such as the hands, feet, perineum, or across joints.

The key question is: Will this burn wound heal spontaneously in a 'reasonable time'? If yes, then all is well and good; if not, with some careful exceptions, surgical treatment delivers the best results with the least pain and the least risk of long-term pain sequelae.

Time to healing

Burns heal by secondary intention from healthy epithelium. This derives from the basement membrane of the epithelium in superficial burns, and from adnexal epithelial structures in shallow dermal burns. There are no such structures surviving in full-thickness burns, and so spontaneous healing of any deep burn bigger than a two-pence piece within a reasonable time span will not occur, therefore, surgery is essential. When spontaneous healing is allowed (very rarely, usually in patients seriously unfit for surgery), healing takes many weeks, the skin quality is poor, patch-up grafting is often still required, scarring is severe and chronic pain is more likely. Burns that may be expected to heal spontaneously include:

- *Superficial burns* affecting only the epidermis will generally heal spontaneously within seven days. There will be peeling and final resolution may take longer, but re-epithelialisation will be confidently apparent within that timescale. The wound will be painful, sometimes exquisitely so, and this pain must be aggressively and appropriately managed by regular multi-modal analgesia with additional, as required, therapy. Chronic pain syndromes are unlikely.
- *Shallow dermal burns* usually have an intact capillary circulation. The skin will blanch on (sterile) digital pressure, and capillary return time will be normal or simply shortened. These wounds heal within two to three weeks with some, but not excessive, scarring. However, between 40% and 60% of these wounds will convert to deep dermal, or even full-thickness wounds under the

influence of the inflammatory response and/or infection in the first 48 to 72 hours. Any wound that has not healed by 10 days should be referred for plastic surgery assessment.

Spontaneous healing is not expected in deep dermal burns. The adnexal structures are more sparse than in shallow dermal burns and unsightly and often unstable scars result. Therefore, grafting at two to three weeks delivers better outcomes in most patients. Asian and African skin types are usually allowed a little more time (a week or two at most) for spontaneous healing, because they are more prone to hypertrophic or keloid scar formation in donor sites as well as the wound itself.

In summary, the appropriate wound management coupled with aggressive pain management, tailored to the type of wound, the stage of healing and any necessary surgical intervention, will minimise negative pain influences and maximise recovery, both physical and psychological.

Lastly, in this context of wound management, it is essential to be vigilant at every patient assessment, be it on the ward or in the clinic, for any change in the wound: redness around, increased swelling, systemic changes such as change in food tolerance or new systemic infection and any shift (usually for the worse) in analgesia requirement. Any/all changes may signify an invasive wound infection, which must be aggressively managed under guidance from a microbiologist with experience of burn wounds. Crucially, even if well managed, an infection usually converts a shallow wound, for which expectant but vigilant management is appropriate, into a deeper wound requiring surgical intervention after the infection has been brought under control.

Specific protocols for procedural pain

A vast number of methods for managing procedural pain in burn care are discussed in the clinical literature. However, the quality of that evidence is variable, generally poor, not least because conducting appropriately controlled studies in this area is difficult — there being just too many variables. Therefore, what follows in this section is a digest based on the experiences of the senior author of this chapter of what works in practice.

Small burns, or larger wounds that have mostly healed, are readily managed by supplements to regular analgesia — additional oral morphine with or without a benzodiazepine being the mainstay. Benzodiazepines are used as adjuncts to opiates in procedural pain to reduce anxiety (Choinière, 2003). A trial of lorazepam showed it was effective in reducing anxiety and opiate requirements in patients with high pain or anxiety scores (Patterson *et al*, 1997). However, in an outpatient setting, benzodiazepine use is usually inappropriate, unless there is somewhere for the patient to sleep it off afterwards. At very least, patients should be encouraged to take their usual analgesia and if they have not done so, it should be given immediately and the procedure delayed to allow time for the medication to be absorbed.

Caution should be exercised when managing nearly-healed wounds, as the pain may be greater than anticipated. Newly-healed scars may be 'angry' and sensitive, and the surrounding normal skin may have become sensitised to touch. Allodynia is fortunately not a common sequel to burn injury, but when it does happen it is very perplexing for the patient: the sense of relief when someone shows that they not only understand but can also explain it, is almost palpable (*Chapter 4*).

Entonox™ (pre-mixed oxygen and nitrous oxide 50:50; British National Formulary [BNF], 2008) is used in initial dressing changes. It is particularly useful as an adjunct to oral analgesia in circumstances where the dressing is mostly comfortable, but with short periods of more extreme soreness. It has a quick onset of action at around 20 seconds and does not cause loss of consciousness or prolonged sedation when self-administered. Furthermore, it can reassure anxious patients with previous negative experiences — discovering that they required less pain control than they thought, helps to improve future confidence. However, there is a risk of megaloblastic anaemia after prolonged exposure that may limit its usefulness for repeated dressing changes. Further studies are required to determine if repeated, daily short exposure to nitrous oxide may further exacerbate the haematological and immunological abnormalities already seen in major burns patients (Pal *et al*, 1997).

Much has been written about non-pharmacological approaches to procedural pain in burns. Hypnosis, virtual reality therapy, cognitive behavioural therapy (CBT), and avoidance and relaxation techniques have all been used to improve pain relief (Pal *et al*, 1997; Choinière, 2003) (*Chapter 9*). For practical purposes, such techniques require time and special expertise that may not be readily available in a busy ward or clinic. There is no doubt, however, that simple distraction works wonders; for adults, the most reassuring distraction and easiest to provide is 'banter'. The nurse or doctor who stays quiet while working unsettles the patient, creating anxiety. You can talk about anything: the weather, recent holidays, what you like to eat. Also, reassuring talk about the wound helps at this time, using the opportunity to educate the patient about what to expect, including that pain is normal and can be treated.

For children, play is invaluable and need not necessarily be simply a distraction. The child can be encouraged to participate in the dressing changes by helping to remove the old dressing, turning it into play (with much splashing if water is being used) (*Chapter 5*). In wards where burn injured children are treated, a separate play area is essential where nothing disagreeable ever happens, including dressing changes.

Patient-controlled analgesia (PCA)

Patient-controlled analgesia (PCA) with morphine or fentanyl is an effective method of pain management for post-operative pain (*Chapter 10*), but has also been used for analgesia during dressing procedures (Prakash *et al*, 2004). The patient has to be physically capable of operating the PCA. This may not be possible if, for example, both the patient's hands are burned. When the patient is asleep and not regularly requesting medication, opioid blood levels will fall and the patient may experience pain on waking. Also, the patient may deliberately under-medicate him or herself to avoid unpleasant side-effects (Choinière, 2003). Nevertheless, the technique has its place.

The fact that oral medication is not always possible or satisfactory is evidenced by a steady trickle of reports of other methods of analgesia delivery. A study in Australia found that patient-controlled intranasal fentanyl (given as a nasal spray) was as effective at controlling the pain of dressing changes and debridement as oral morphine (Finn *et al*, 2004). Fentanyl-containing lollipops have been used successfully for analgesia delivery in children (Choinière, 2003). Non-invasive analgesia lessens the risk of infection and may be important where intravenous access is difficult or impossible.

Intravenous infusions

For major dressing changes, standard opioids may not be the best choice for procedural pain as they are relatively slow to act and excess sedation may continue long after the procedure has ended. Short-acting opioids, such as fentanyl, given intravenously may be more suitable, but more effective in practice is the use of sedatives and analgesics by continuous infusion.

Propofol and alfentanil by infusion can, with experience, be titrated to provide excellent sedation without loss of airway (Gallagher *et al*, 2000). Remifentanil is a new, very short-acting opioid, which can be used with propofol, but is also increasingly used alone as it gives profound analgesia while retaining consciousness and a degree of cooperation. In all such techniques, the margin between adequate sedation and general anaesthesia is so narrow that anaesthesia expertise and monitoring are essential. Remifentanil is so short-acting that it provides no residual analgesia after it is stopped, so another means of ensuring continued analgesia must be provided before the end of the procedure.

Ketamine

Ketamine was developed as a general anaesthetic, but is used mainly in developing countries where specialist expertise is hard to come by, or for induction in patients who are seriously compromised (for example, bleeding aortic aneurysm). Ketamine is a potent analgesic and is therefore still used to provide analgesia and sedation for dressing changes; it can also reduce opioid requirements when long use is associated with tachyphylaxis in sedated patients in intensive care. However, it is associated with a 5–30% incidence of emergence delirium reactions, particularly in the elderly (Patterson *et al*, 2004). These may be minimised but not entirely eliminated by the concurrent use of benzodiazepines. Nevertheless, it remains a useful agent for dressing changes in small children. In particular, when low doses are used carefully as a sedative-analgesic. These children seem not to experience hallucinations, or perhaps are not bothered by them.

General anaesthesia

There are circumstances, e.g: initial aggressive wound debridement on admission particularly in children; the first dressing after graft surgery; and repeated dressing of extensive burns, when general anaesthesia may be the only means of achieving satisfactory pain control for a non-operative procedure. Because general anaesthetic agents have a depressive effect on bone marrow and the immune response mechanisms already diminished by the burn injury, and because they inhibit nutrition intake, their use for non-operative procedures is kept to a minimum, and the patient is 'weaned' onto other analgesia regimens as soon as possible. Adequate analgesia must be established during recovery.

Local anaesthesia

Donor site analgesia can be achieved by topical application of local anaesthetic (0.5% bupivacaine or 2% lidocaine mixed 1:1 with aqueous gel, or lidocaine 2% spray) before the dressing is applied (Norman and Judkins, 2004). The possibility that absorption from this site may risk systemic toxicity has been explored in one reassuring study of small donor sites (Bulmer and Duckett, 1985); but Patterson *et al* (2004) mention (but do not reference) reports of seizures linked to systemic absorption at the open wound site; this question would seem to remain an open one.

Nerve blocks
Where burns are restricted to specific areas, such as the arm or the leg, nerve blocks are an option for procedural pain. They have the advantage of relatively quick onset, may reduce opioid requirements and therefore side-effects, and can provide complete analgesia for several hours. Drawbacks include the time taken to give the block and the risk of infection. A small study ($n = 20$) at a centre which usually harvests skin for grafts from the medial or lateral upper thigh found that a femoral nerve block of 0.2% bupivacaine or ropivocaine was effective in reducing opiate requirements, although opiate side-effects were not reduced (Cuignet *et al*, 2004). Another study of 100 patients found that using a nerve block during the harvesting procedure itself provided adequate analgesia (Gupta *et al*, 2007).

Conclusion

Burns are common and extremely painful, yet the literature concurs that burn pain management is often inadequate. Burn pain management is complex, with several different types of pain to manage and many treatment options. To achieve a high level of pain control, pain must be regularly and adequately assessed and analgesia tailored to the individual's needs and psychological state.

While there is data in the literature focusing on many different aspects of burn pain management, a large proportion is either case reports or clinical trials with sample sizes too small for the results to be considered significant. This may be due to the small numbers of inpatients with comparable injuries treated at individual burn centres. The majority of studies acknowledge this and recommend further research. Multi-centre or national studies may be necessary to achieve a significant sample size.

References

Aaron LA, Patterson DR, Finch CP, Carrougher GJ, Heimbach DM (2001) The utility of a burn specific measure of pain anxiety to prospectively predict pain and function: a comparative analysis. *Burns* 27(4): 329–34

Atchison NE, Osgood PF, Carr DB, Szyfelbein SK (1991) Pain during burn dressing change in children: relationship to burn area, depth and analgesic regimens. *Pain* 47(1): 41–5

Barret JP, Dziewulski P, Ramzy PI, Wolf SE, Desai MH, Herndon DN (2000) Biobrane versus 1% silver sulfadiazine in second-degree pediatric burns. *Plast Reconstr Surg* 105(1): 62–5

British Burn Association (2001) *Standards and Strategy for Burn Care: A review of burn care in the British Isles.* British Burn Association, London

British National Formulary (2008) British National Formulary (56). BMA & Royal Pharmaceutical Society of Great Britain, London

Brooks JP, Malic CC, Judkins KC (2008) Scratching the surface — managing the itch associated with burns: A review of current knowledge. *Burns* 34(6): 751–60

Bulmer JN, Duckett AC (1985) Absorption of lignocaine through split-skin donor sites. *Anaesthesia* 40(8): 808–9

Byers JF, Bridges S, Kijek J, LaBorde P (2001) Burn patients' pain and anxiety experiences. *J Burn Care Rehabil* 22(2): 144–9

Choinière M (2003) Pain of burns. In: Melzack R, Wall PD, eds. *Handbook of Pain Management: a clinical companion to Wall and Melzack's 'Textbook of Pain'.* Churchill Livingstone, Edinburgh: 591–601

Cuignet O, Pirson J, Boughrouph J, Duville D (2004) The efficacy of continuous fascia iliaca compartment block for pain management in burn patients undergoing skin grafting procedures. *Anesth Analg* 98(4): 1077–81

Cuignet O, Pirson J, Soudon O, Zizi M (2007) Effects of gabapentin on morphine consumption and pain in severely burned patients. *Burns* 33(1): 81–6

Dauber A, Osgood PF, Breslau AJ, Vernon HL, Carr DB (2002) Chronic persistent pain after severe burns: a survey of 358 burn survivors. *Pain Med* 3(1): 6–17

Dearden C, Donnelly J, Dunlop M, Dunlop M, Higgins M, Tieney E (2001) Traumatic wounds: the management of superficial and partial thickness burns. *Nurs Times* 97(48): 53–5

Finn J, Wright J, Fong J, et al (2004) A randomised crossover trial of patient-controlled intranasal fentanyl and oral morphine for procedural wound care in adult patients with burns. *Burns* 30(3): 262–8

Franulic A, Gonzalez X, Trucco M, Vallejos F (1996) Emotional and psychosocial factors in burn patients during hospitalization. *Burns* 22(8): 618–22

Gallagher G, Rae CP, Kenny GN, Kinsella J (2000) The use of a target-controlled infusion of alfentanil to provide analgesia for burn dressing changes. A dose finding study. *Anaesthesia* 55(12): 1159–63

Gupta A, Bhandari PS, Shrivastava P (2007) A study of regional nerve blocks and local anaesthetic creams (Prilox) for donor sites in burn patients. *Burns* 33(1): 87–91

Hettiaratchy S, Dziewulski P (2004) ABC of burns: pathophysiology and types of burns. *Br Med J* 328(7453): 1427–9

Hettiaratchy S, Papini R (2004) Initial management of a major burn: II — assessment and resuscitation. *Br Med J* 329(7457): 101–3

Jonsson CE, Holmsten A, Dahlstrom L, Jonsson K (1998) Background pain in burn patients: routine measurement and recording of pain intensity in a burn unit. *Burns* 24(5): 448–54

Latarjet J, Choinière M (1995) Pain in burn patients. *Burns* 21(5): 344–8

McCaffery M, Pasero C (1999) *Pain: Clinical manual.* 2nd edn. Mosby, London

Melzack R, Wall PD (2003) *Handbook of pain management: a clinical companion to Wall and Melzack's 'Textbook of Pain'.* Churchill Livingstone, Edinburgh

Mikkelsen S, Jorgensen H, Larsen PS, Brennum J, Dahl JB (2000) Effect of oral ketamine on secondary hyperalgesia, thermal and mechanical pain thresholds, and sedation in humans. *Regional Anaesth Pain Med* 25(5): 452–8

Norman A, Judkins K (2004) Pain in the patient with burns. *Contin Educ Anaesth Crit Care Pain* 4(2): 57–61

Pal SK, Cortiella J, Herndon D (1997) Adjunctive methods of pain control in burns. *Burns* 23(5): 404–12

Papini R (2004) Management of burn injuries of various depths. *Br Med J* 329(7458): 158–60

Patterson DR, Everett JJ, Bombardier CH, *et al* (1993) Psychological effects of severe burn injuries. *Psychol Bull* 113(2): 362–78

Patterson DR, Ptacek JT, Carrougher GJ, Sharar SR (1997) Lorazepam as an adjunct to opioid analgesics in the treatment of burn pain. *Pain* 72(3): 367–74

Patterson DR, Hofland HW, Espey K, Sharar S (2004) Pain management. *Burns* 30(8): A10–15

Perry S, Heidrich G (1982) Management of pain during debridement: a survey of U.S. burn units. *Pain* 13(3): 267–80

Prakash S, Fatima T, Pawar M (2004) Patient-controlled analgesia with fentanyl for burn dressing changes. *Anesth Analg* **99**(2): 552–5

Taal LA, Faber AW (1997) Post-traumatic stress, pain and anxiety in adult burn victims. *Burns* **23**(7–8): 545–9

Wachtel TL, Berry CC, Wachtel EE, Frank HA (2000) The inter-rater reliability of estimating the size of burns from various burn area chart drawings. *Burns* **26**(2): 156–70

World Health Organization (2008) WHO's pain ladder. WHO, Geneva. Available online at: www.who.int/cancer/palliative/painladder/en/ [accessed 8 October 2008]

CHAPTER 8

PHARMACOLOGICAL METHODS OF PAIN CONTROL

Michelle Briggs, Tarnia Taverner and Barry Strickland Hodge

Pain associated with wounds, represents a key threat to healing, as people in pain are unable to participate fully in activities to promote healing such as exercise, dressing changes or compression therapy (Briggs and Flemming, 2007; Mallet, 1999). As Persoon *et al* (2004) state: 'It is quite possible that reducing pain levels and improving mobility capacity will have a positive effect on wound healing'. It is important therefore to have an integrated approach which focuses on pain management parallel to wound healing decisions when caring for people with wounds. This is especially important when wounds last longer than a few weeks. It is possible that the longer someone is left in pain without effective treatment, the greater the risk to that person in terms of healing, psychological well-being and social isolation (Persoon *et al*, 2004). In other areas, effective pain management has been shown to have a positive impact on healing. McGuire *et al* (2006) undertook a five-week prospective study investigating the impact of effective pain management on wound healing. They found patients who had untreated pain were significantly associated with subsequent delayed healing.

Despite this, there is evidence that pharmacological interventions to reduce pain are under-used for people with wound pain (Hew de Laat *et al*, 2005). For example, in a study by Szor and Bourguignon (1999), 75% of the participants reported moderate to severe pain as a result of pressure ulceration, but only 6% had an analgesic prescription. In an Italian wound care study ($n = 381$), only 2/3 received analgesia and only 23% were prescribed pain relief as recommended by the World Health Organization (WHO) (66% used as required analgesia rather than regular medication) and there was no report of adjuvant analgesic use for neuropathic pain (Guarnera *et al*, 2007). In a study by Heinen *et al* (2006) (*n* = 141), a similar picture is seen — 50% of leg ulcer patients in pain either did not use analgesics or used them only occasionally.

Addressing the source of pain

Being an internal sensation, it can be difficult for healthcare professionals to fully understand what patients are really experiencing when they describe pain. If a person has a wound there are a number of processes which could be the origin of the pain. These processes could exist in isolation or in combination. Pharmacological methods need to address the pain at its source if they are to be effective.

Pain of predominantly nociceptive origin

Most commonly, pain is generated from the wound inflammatory process . This is nociceptive pain and could be described as 'normal or ordinary' pain. It is the pain most people would recognise. It occurs when a person injures themselves and healthy tissue is damaged. This is a person's normal pain response to injury and is usually time limited. This type of pain is likely to respond to the WHO analgesic ladder (WHO, 2008).

WHO ladder step 1: mild pain or pain score of 1–3 (0–10 scale)

Paracetamol is an analgesic and antipyretic drug that acts via a central site of action (Courade *et al*, 2001; Muth-Selbach *et al*, 1999). Paracetamol can be used alone or as an adjunct to other analgesics. Paracetamol is the first drug of choice for many chronic painful conditions (WHO, 2008); it is also the National Kidney Foundation's drug choice for patients with renal disease (Ruoff, 1998). Paracetamol is effective for mild to moderate pain, but a stronger analgesic is required for pain that is described as moderate to severe (WHO, 2008).

Non-steroidal anti-inflammatory drugs (NSAIDs)
These have analgesic, anti-inflammatory and/or antipyretic properties. They should be used for mild to moderate pain associated with injury or inflammation, they can also be given in combination with opioid

medications for the treatment of severe pain (Manning and Richer, 2003).

The authors are aware of only one randomised controlled trial of oral aspirin (an NSAID) for chronic venous leg ulcers (Layton *et al*, 1994). Unfortunately, they only studied the effect on healing and no pain scores were recorded. After four months, ulcer healing was achieved in 38% of the aspirin group and 0% of the placebo group. The authors attributed this to the anticoagulant properties of aspirin. A major issue, however, when considering using aspirin or NSAIDS is balancing their beneficial effects with their adverse event profile. For example, NSAIDS have at times been avoided in people with wounds for fear that they would interfere with wound healing (Snaith, 1992; Bush and Bonney, 1992).

NSAIDs work by inhibiting cyclo-oxygenase (COX 1, COX 2, or both) and reduce the production of prostaglandins and leukotrienes. Prostaglandins and other cyclo-oxygenase products sensitise peripheral nerve endings and amplify the effects of other inflammatory mediators such as bradykinin (Carr and Goudas, 1999). Hence, NSAIDS reduce pain by removing some prostaglandins. However, due to this inhibition many adverse effects are associated with NSAIDs.

COX 1 is thought to be responsible for the synthesis of prostaglandins in areas where they have a protective function (e.g. renal medulla and gastric mucosa). COX 1 assists with the homeostatic control in the kidney, gut, mucosa, smooth muscle, platelets and endothelium (Manning and Richer, 2003). In the gastrointestinal tract, prostaglandins decrease acid secretion and increase the production of mucus and bicarbonate (Hersh, 2000). In the renal vasculature, prostaglandins have a vasodilatory activity that helps maintain renal perfusion and function. COX 1 is the group of prostaglandins involved in normal physiological activity, whereas COX 2 produces prostaglandins involved in inflammation and pain.

There are well documented potential risks associated with the use of NSAIDs, especially in older people (Bandolier, 2008). NSAIDs are associated with a number of important adverse effects (see below). These include effects on the kidney, exacerbating asthma in some people and problems in the gastrointestinal tract. NSAIDs also cause gastric erosions that can become ulcers. The burden of NSAID adverse effects in the UK is significant, there are approximately 25 million prescriptions written for NSAIDs in the UK annually which lead to 12,000 NSAID-related hospital admissions and approximately 2,600 deaths (Bandolier, 2008). Coulling (2007) suggests a useful mnemonic of BRAGHH — never give NSAIDs if there is evidence of:

- bleeding
- renal impairment
- aspirin sensitive asthmatic
- gastric irritation
- hypotension
- heart failure (*Table 8.1*).

Despite these statistics, it must be acknowledged that NSAIDs are effective analgesics, bringing a huge benefit to many people who use them. The recommendation from Bandolier is that the risks are age-related, with high risk associated with people 75 years and over (Blower *et al*, 1997). The leg ulceration literature has only one qualitative study where the use of diclofenac is mentioned (Guarnera *et al*, 2007), there is no quantitative study investigating the use of oral NSAIDs to manage the pain associated with chronic wounds. However, there are some studies which test a new product containing topical ibuprofen.

Topical ibuprofen

There are studies investigating the use of ibuprofen as a topical agent in the form of Biatain Ibu (Coloplast A/S), which is a foam dressing that releases low dose ibuprofen. Jorgensen *et al* (2006) carried out a single blinded cross-over trial using a pre-treatment period of two placebo dressings, a test treatment period of five active foam dressings containing ibuprofen, and a washout period with two placebo dressings. The patients were aged between 58 and 89 years (mean=82.9), all had venous leg ulcers and most of them had had leg ulcers before. The Biatain Ibu treatment correlated with a decrease in pain intensity scores from seven in the pre-treatment period to approximately 2.5 in the Biatain Ibu phase. Patients were also assessed for blood plasma levels of ibuprofen, and blood serum samples showed no ibuprofen. However, only 10 patients were included in the trial and no report of oral analgesics was given

A further study to investigate the use of topical ibuprofen, used case series methodology and collected qualitative as well as quantitative data. This study had small numbers (*n*=10) of five men and five women. Participants were treated with the foam dressing releasing ibuprofen for six dressing changes, followed by a non pain-relieving

Table 8.1: Contraindications of non-steroidal anti-inflammatory drugs	
Bleeding	Platelet adhesiveness is reduced caution in those on anticoagulant therapy or with bleeding problems, e.g haemophilia
Renal impairment	Care in those with high creatinine, hypovolaemia, low urine output or on Angiotensin converting enzyme (ACE) inhibitors
Aspirin, sensitive asthmatic	10% of asthmatics are sensitive to NSAIDs
Gastric irritation	Care if history of gastric ulceration. Patients at risk may need a gastro-protective agent (a proton pump inhibitor – omeprazole or lansoprazole)
Hypotension	NSAIDs compromise renal perfusion particularly in hypotensive states
Heart failure	May worsen due to NSAIDs induced fluid retention

foam dressing in the non-active treatment phase. When treated with the topical ibuprofen-containing dressing, patient pain decreased and then increased one week after the study when the treatment had discontinued (Flanagan *et al*, 2007).

A further three trials have added to the evidence for this product (Sibbald *et al*, 2006; Gottrup *et al*, 2007; Domenech *et al*, 2008). The most recent study was a well designed open pragmatic randomised controlled trial of 184 local wound care centres in 12 countries across Europe, Israel and Canada. A total of 853 people were recruited to receive either Biatain Ibu or local best practice. Anyone who had a wound with moderate to severe levels of exudate was included in the sample. However, it is worth noting that infected wounds; larger wounds than the dressing could accommodate; wounds with exposed bones, muscles or tendons; grade 1, 3 and 4 pressure ulcers and grades 3, 4, 5 diabetic foot ulcers were all excluded from the sample. Those with any contraindication to NSAIDs were also excluded.

The primary endpoint was level of pain relief achieved on a scale of 0–4 and the secondary endpoint was the reduction in the intensity of persistent pain from day 0 to day 7. The research team used intention to treat analysis and demonstrated that the study had sufficient power to detect a difference in the selected outcomes. Both the primary and secondary endpoints favoured the treatment group.

The treatment group experienced a mean reduction in pain intensity of 3.7 versus 1.5 in the local best practice group after seven days of treatment.

Although the results from this study are promising, there are limitations as the trial dressing was not blinded to participants or trial assessors, which means people may have been biased toward the new dressing. Also, without knowing what local best practice is, it is difficult to make a considered judgement about how effective Biatain Ibu is in comparison. There is evidence that pain management for people with wounds is inadequate in many places (Persoon, 2004; Hew De Laat, 2005). Therefore, in some centres, Biatain Ibu could have been compared to regular use of the WHO analgesic ladder, and in others it could have been compared to no other pain relief. It would have been useful to have more detail of the concomitant oral analgesic intake and compare this between groups. It is worth noting that despite being asked not to alter their analgesic medication, statistically significantly more people in the Biatain Ibu group chose to reduce their intake compared to the local best practice group (39% versus 19%).

Gottrupp *et al* (2007) studied 122 patients for a slightly longer period (six weeks) and their results echoed Domenech *et al* (2008). They randomised 62 leg ulcer patients to receive Biatain Ibu and 60 patients to receive a similar dressing. The issue of bias was addressed as this trial was also double blind. People were once again excluded if they had a contraindication to NSAIDs, infected wounds, did not have moderate or heavily exuding wounds. Patients were also excluded if they 'had painful ulcers that had been resistant to analgesic treatment over the last six months'. They assessed persistent pain relief on a five-point scale (no relief 0, slight 1, moderate 2, lots 3, complete 4), but then dichotomised the data to pain relief yes or no in the final analysis. Therefore, while the results showed that 46/62 achieved pain relief in the Biatain Ibu group and 35/60 achieved pain relief in the foam in week 1, it not possible to assess the magnitude of the relief obtained. Although the pain scores do indicate a shift of 2.7 in favour of the Biatain Ibu group (from 6.8 to 4.1), compared to 2.0 with the foam dressing alone (6.6 to 4.6).

Biatain Ibu may be a useful addition for some people, but it would seem that wounds need to have moderate exudate to activate the ibuprofen, so for those people with wounds that have low exudate it may not be an option. Also, while studies of a few weeks' duration may be sufficient to test the effect of the dressings' ability to relieve pain, it is not sufficient to test the impact on healing. Domenech *et al* (2008) suggest that because there were few dressing-related events reported during that week, that this indicates that the dressing safety and tolerability was good. It would be more prudent to suggest we need long-term outcome studies to indicate this. There were 31 adverse events in Gottrup *et al*'s study (2007), 21 in the NSAID group and 10 in the control. This was not statistically significant and while Gottrup *et al* suggest that, 'other clinical studies on the ibuprofen foam including more than 373 patients have not detected any cases of allergic or contact dermatitis as adverse reactions', this is still a small number of patients and the effects of long-term use of topical ibuprofen is unknown.

WHO ladder step 2: moderate pain or pain score of 3–6 (on 0–10 scale)

Opium contains approximately 25 different alkaloids, only two of these have any analgesic action — morphine (10% by weight of opium) and codeine (0.5% by weight). These naturally occurring substances are called opiates. An opioid is any compound (natural or synthetic), which has pharmacological activity at an opioid receptor. The activity of these compounds can be reversed by an opioid antagonist (for example, naloxone). Codeine is a low potency opioid and is the drug recommended at stage two of the analgesic ladder (WHO, 2008) for mild to moderate pain. If pain relief is insufficient with paracetamol alone, codeine may be added as an adjunct. Combining two different analgesics can avoid increasing the dose of either drug, thus reducing the likelihood of side-effects from either medication (Helme and Katz, 2003). A systematic review investigating the use of paracetamol with or without codeine confirmed that codeine 60 mg produced worthwhile additional pain relief (Moore *et al*, 1997). Tramadol could be recommended in this weak opioids section (Woo *et al*, 2008), although there is a caution associated with use of tramadol which is the possibility of convulsions at high doses. An Australian study found that of the 97 confirmed new-onset seizures, eight were associated with tramadol, and that in the author's 'First seizure clinic', tramadol was the most frequently suspected cause of provoked seizures (Labate, 2005). Moreover, the risk increases in older people, as the elimination half-life can be prolonged.

WHO ladder step 3: severe pain or score of 7–10

Morphine is the 'gold standard' opioid. It is the most commonly used and is the standard against which all other opioids are tested (Heffernan and Rowbotham, 2003). It is metabolised by hepatic conjugation and its major metabolites are morphine 6-glucuronide (M6G) and morphine 3-glucuronide. M6G is an active metabolite and is responsible for a significant amount of pharmacological activity (Vermeire and Remon, 1999). Accumulation of M6G may contribute to analgesia and μ receptor related side-effects, such as sedation (Macintyre *et al*, 2003). Age rather than weight should be a predictor to the amount of opioid given, morphine and fentanyl requirements are known to decrease with age. A number of studies have shown that the average morphine requirements of a 70-year-old are only 32–38% of the average doses required by a 20-year-old patient (Macintyre and Jarvis, 1996). The effects of morphine can be countered with opioid antagonists such as naloxone and naltrexone. Fentanyl is a powerful opioid analgesic, approximately 100 times more potent than morphine. The usual routes of administration are intravenous, subcutaneous, spinal, transdermal and transmucosal (Ribeiro and Zeppetella, 2002).

Transdermal fentanyl (durogesic/duragesic)
Fentanyl patches work by releasing fentanyl into body fats, which then slowly release the drug into the blood stream over 48 to 72 hours, allowing for long-lasting relief from pain. Rate of absorption is dependent on a number of factors, including: body temperature, skin type, amount of body fat, and placement of the patch. The different delivery systems used by different manufacturers will also affect individual rates of absorption. Under normal circumstances, the analgesic effect of fentanyl patches begins within 8 and 12 hours, thus fentanyl patches are often prescribed with another opioid (such as morphine sulfate) for breakthrough pain. Due to absorption rates being unpredictable in older people because of differences in body temperature and subcutaneous fat and water, transdermal fentanyl patches should be avoided (Gloth, 2001). Although the fentanyl patch may be useful in a situation where medication cannot be administered orally, an opioid-naïve person should not be started on a dose more than 25 micrograms an hour. It must also be noted that after removal of a patch, there is a subcutaneous reservoir of active drug in the serum, the half-life of which is approximately 18 hours (Gloth, 2001).

Transmucosal fentanyl

Recently, research using intranasal or inhaled fentanyl have been reported (e.g. Zeppetella, 2001; Borland, 2005), however it is oral (buccal) transmucosal delivery that has attracted the most interest (Ribeiro and Zeppetella, 2002). A flavoured-lollipop of fentanyl citrate mixed with inert fillers on a stick was introduced under the brand name of Actiq, becoming the first quick-acting formulation of fentanyl for use with breakthrough chronic pain.

More recently, fentanyl has been further developed into an effervescent tablet for buccal absorption much like the Actiq lollipop; a buccal spray device for fast-acting relief and other delivery methods which are currently in development. The tablet is a berry-flavoured lozenge on a stick which is swabbed on the mucosal surfaces inside the mouth — inside of the cheeks, under and on the tongue and gums — to release the fentanyl quickly into the system. It is most effective when the lozenge is consumed in 15 minutes. Patients find it takes 10–15 minutes to use all of one lozenge, and those with a dry mouth may not be able to use this route.

Long-acting or sustained-release preparations are the most appropriate types of opioids to use for the management of chronic non-malignant pain, because of their single or twice-daily usage and stable blood concentrations, as a consequence of their more predictable pharmacokinetics (Goucke and Graziotti, 2003).

Short-acting opioids are more appropriate for moderate to severe episodic pain, for example, pain at dressing changes. Assuming that the patient is not opioid tolerant, it is prudent to monitor for somnolence and hypoxemia if using fentanyl for procedural pain (see Aronoff, 2005 or Hofman, 2006 for guidance) The recommendation from many is to start the opioids using a low dose and escalate slowly, while titrating the amount required to the individual patient (American Geriatrics Society [AGS], 1998; Gloth, 2001). The British Pain Society published recommendations for the appropriate use of opioids for persistent non-cancer pain which provides useful information and is available to download (www.britishpainsociety.org/book_opioid_main.pdf).

Possible side-effects of opioids

Nausea, vomiting, itching and somnolence are the most common side-effects from opioids. More serious problems include respiratory depression, weight gain, weight loss, and hormonal effects such as reduced adrenal function, reduced sexual function and infertility in long-term opioid use (British Pain Society, 2004).

Respiratory depression

The risk of respiratory depression when oral opioids are being used for chronic pain is reduced when appropriate doses are used and they are titrated against the pain scores.

Nausea and vomiting

The likelihood of opioids causing nausea and vomiting is uncertain, some of the effect may come from stimulation of opioid receptors at the chemo-receptor trigger zone in the medulla (McQuay, 1999). The nausea should resolve within the first few days of starting opioids and decrease with time in the majority of patients. In some cases it is recommended that an alternative opioid be tried.

Constipation

Constipation is a side-effect of all opioids, it occurs as a result of opioid binding to the gastrointestinal (GI) tract, leading to decreased peristalsis, reduced intestinal secretions, and increased re-absorption of fluids from the colon. This is a side-effect that requires particular attention for older people. It is recommended that upon initiation of opioids certain measures should be taken. Use of a laxative, adequate fluid intake, ambulation and exercise should be encouraged (Gloth, 1996; Maxwell, 2000). Unlike other opioid side-effects, tolerance to the opioid does not prevent constipation.

Itching

It is thought that opioid induced pruritus may result from action on the opioid receptor (Ballantyne *et al*, 1988). Due to this action, antihistamines may not be effective, it is also important to acknowledge that antihistamines are likely to cause side-effects in the older person (Macintyre *et al*, 2003). Although itching should subside after initiation of opioids, it may persist and preclude continuation of the drug (British Pain Society, 2004).

Neurological and psychological side-effects

These are side-effects such as sedation, loss of concentration and ability to drive. Cognitive dysfunction is more likely in the early treatment of pain with opioids; studies suggest that regular use of opioids is much less likely to result in impairment of psychomotor or cognitive process than healthy volunteers. In a study investigating oral opioid therapy in patients with chronic non-malignant pain, it was shown that participants did suffer from fatigue, nausea, vomiting and dizziness, however, these reactions only occurred in the initial titration phase and once stability of dose was obtained, adverse events subsided (Zenz *et al*, 1992). The study also found that if opioid therapy provided adequate pain relief, patients' performance was enhanced because the obstacle that the pain represented was no longer the central concern of their daily life. Thus, they state that long-term use of opioid analgesics in chronic pain does not lead to anguish or isolation, but to an improvement in performance, and often opens the way for additional measures to treat pain such as physiotherapy. In another study it was found that patients with non-malignant chronic pain taking long-acting opioids showed significant improvements on a measure of psychomotor speed and sustained attention. The authors suggested that long-acting opioids can improve mood and do not impair cognitive functioning in patients with chronic non-malignant pain (Haythornthwaite *et al*, 1998).

Topical morphine

The discovery of opiate receptors on peripheral nerve terminals by Stein (1995) has lead to the use of opioids topically in wounds. This has been reported in the literature but only in case series studies.

Ballas (2002) reported a case of using topical opioids. The report was with a 38-year-old woman with a sickle cell leg ulcer. Her pain score was 10 on a 0–10 scale, and she was taking 16–18 tablets of oxycodone per day with little relief. In an effort to relieve the pain, one oxycodone tablet was dissolved in 2 ml of water and applied directly to the wound. This gave almost immediate relief and reduced her pain score to 0. Oxycodone consumption reduced to 0–2 tablets per day. Others have reported case studies with findings that support this in the area of palliative care (Back and Finlay, 1995; Twillman, 1999; Krajnik *et al*, 1999; Flock, 2000). In these cases, morphine or diamorphine were used with intrasite gel (a hydrogel wound preparation).

Between 2003 and 2004 a randomised controlled trial attempted to address the question of effectiveness (Vernaissaire *et al*, 2005). Twenty leg ulcer or pressure ulcer patients were randomised to receive either morphine in Intrasite® gel (Smith and Nephew Healthcare) covered with Comfeel®(Coloplast), or placebo Intrasite gel covered with Comfeel. The groups were indistinguishable. Each group received WHO level 2 pain treatment as described above (codeine, tramadol or dextropropoxyphene), and level 3 'rescue analgesia' if required (morphine sulphate). Unfortunately, despite 24 being recruited, only 14 completed the study (six withdrew consent with no reason being given and two left due to failure to achieve pain relief, one with maceration and one with infection). The degree of pain relief achieved was not statistically significantly different between the groups. The study was limited by poor recruitment and retention and the author called for more multicentre trials in this area. Flock (2003) also suggested that a larger trial was required following the results of her randomised, double blind, crossover trial of 13 patients with pressure ulcers in palliative care. Again, while 13 patients were recruited, only seven completed the study. Two patients died before randomisation, one patient developed an acute confusional state, and the other three died during the course of the study. The author suggested that topical diamorphine was significantly better than placebo, but acknowledged that the high attrition rate was a problem which is common in palliative care studies (Flock, 2003). A larger study would be required to confirm these findings.

Several questions need answering before topical opioids can be recommended for use in chronic wounds. The morphine absorption via a chronic open wound is unknown. An experimental study where morphine was applied to the skin of healthy volunteers with the epidermis removed showed a bioavailability of 75% (Westerling *et al*, 1994). Also, it is not clear which opioid is the first-line choice; oxycodone, morphine and diamorphine have all produced positive results. Equally, the best carrier gel is not clear and there is the question of whether a slow-release formulation may be a better alternative. The impact on wound healing would also need to be investigated if the intervention were to have clinical utility outside the palliative care field. There has been some preliminary work examining the effect of topically applied opioids on the healing of open ischaemic wounds in rats which suggested that opioids accelerate wound healing (Poonawala *et al*, 2005). This remains an interesting area for future research.

Pain of predominantly neuropathic origin

Neuropathic pain is caused by damage to the nervous system and it has been estimated that almost half of the neuropathies come from either trauma, inflammation or infection (Gatchel *et al*, 2007). This sort of pain is extraordinary pain feeling like burning, shooting, stabbing, or electric shocks. Injured or damaged nerves can heal without causing pain, but sometimes (and it is not always possible to predict who this will happen to) these nerves can become excitable and start to fire off pain impulses from the site of the nerve damage long after the surrounding tissues have healed. This is part of the explanation behind phantom limb pain.

Neuropathic pain has been shown to be prevalent in chronic wound populations (Briggs *et al*, 2007). Therefore, it is important that it is recognised and treated.

Anticonvulsants (of which gabapentin is one) are a group of medicines commonly used for treating 'fits' or epilepsy, but they are also effective for treating this type of pain as they are thought to 'damp down' nerve activity. Approximately two-thirds of patients who take either carbamazepine or gabapentin can expect to achieve good pain relief if the pain is chronic. However, there is no evidence of benefit in acute pain (Wiffen *et al*, 2005). Although gabapentin is effective, its inter-subject variability and non-linear pharmacokinetics make it sometimes difficult to predict the appropriate dose, or which patients are likely to achieve a meaningful clinical response (Rice and Maton, 2001). Pregabalin was given UK approval for use in neuropathic pain in 2004 (Lyrica® [Pfizer]).

Antidepressants, for example, amitriptyline, or more recently, venlafaxine, are offered to people for neuropathic pain. A systematic review noted that at least one-third of patients with neuropathic pain who took traditional antidepressants obtained moderate pain relief or better, and venlafaxine had similar effectiveness to traditional antidepressants. However, approximately one-fifth of those who take these medicines for pain discontinue the therapy due to adverse effects (Saarto and Wiffen, 2007). A modified version of the WHO analgesic ladder for use in leg ulcer clinics has been developed by Hofman *et al* in Oxford (2006), which incorporates the use of these drugs.

Treatment-related pain

In a recent international survey where practitioners from 11 European countries were questioned, the practitioners surveyed indicated that pain at dressing changes was common and was caused by dressing adherence and wound cleansing (Moffatt, 2002). Another wound treatment is sharp debridement of slough and necrotic tissue. This is advocated by some clinicians as the fastest way of achieving a clean wound which, in turn, is thought to improve healing. It is thought that debridement reduces odour, lowers the risk of infection and improves the result of skin grafting (Vanscheidt, 2001; Blanke and Hallern, 2003). However, debridement is not without risks; it is an extremely painful procedure (Hansson, 1993) and patients often ask clinicians to stop before the debridement is complete because they are unable to tolerate the resulting pain (Enander Malmros, 1990; Lok *et al*, 1999). In addition, sharp debridement may delay wound healing as there is a risk of damaging healthy tissue and underlying blood vessels (Vanscheidt, 2001). Compression therapy has also been recognised as painful and people have difficulty tolerating it, especially in the first few weeks (Briggs and Closs, 2006; Edwards, 2003). Therefore, pre-emptive analgesia before an anticipated painful event is likely to help more people to tolerate the iatrogenic pain.

Local anaesthetics (LA)

The use of EMLA cream to manage pain associated with debridement of leg ulcers has been investigated. EMLA is an emulsion in which the oil phase is a mixture of 2.5% lidocaine and 2.5% prilocaine, it works by targeting the free nerve endings, preventing the initiation and transmission of nerve impulses. EMLA cream has been effective in relieving the pain associated with chronic leg ulcers. In a systematic review carried out by Briggs and Nelson (Briggs and Nelson, 2003) six randomised controlled trials of EMLA versus 'placebo' or 'no anaesthesia' were included (Holm *et al*, 1990; Johnson and Repper, 1992; Holst and Kristofferson, 1998; Agrifoglio *et al*, 2000; Enander *et al*, 2000; Rosenthal *et al*, 2001). Length of cream application and plasma concentration was investigated by (Holst and Kristofferson, 1998; Enander *et al*, 2000). This review was restricted to randomised controlled trials. Five out of six studies that were included in the review reported a statistically significant reduction in pain when EMLA 5% was used topically, and applied for 30–45 minutes under occlusion before debridement of the leg ulcer was carried out. EMLA was shown to decrease the incidence of post-debridement pain and reduced the time needed to obtain a clean ulcer. The meta-analysis results suggested that people with venous leg ulcers should expect their post-debridement pain to be reduced by 20 mm on a 100 mm visual analogue scale (VAS). EMLA is currently approved as a topical anaesthetic for the debridement of leg ulcers in Belgium, Denmark, Finland, France, Germany, Netherlands, Norway, Portugal, Spain, Sweden and Switzerland (Blanke and Hallern, 2003).

Reports of toxicity associated with topical use of local anaesthetics have mainly been observed with their application to mucosal membranes leading to rapid absorption, and the application of lidocaine gel to burn wounds causing seizures in children (Pal *et al*, 1997). Blanke and Hallern (2003) concur that the use of EMLA on wounds in children has not been well studied and there are safety concerns. They report a six-year follow-up study of 1084 patients using EMLA for debridement in their department. Of the 1084 patients, 312 had leg ulcers and 384 had pressure ulcers, the remaining sample comprised burns, abcesses, diabetic ulcers and surgical wounds. Ulcers sizes ranged from 5–360 cm^2. There were no cases of local anaesthetic toxicity (central nervous system or cardiovascular) or evidence of prilocaine overdose (cyanosis, nausea, vomiting). The incidence of burning was 1.1% . Unfortunately, healing rates are not reported. A concern with using topical local anaesthetics for the management of pain associated with leg ulcers over a long period of time is the unknown potential effect that these local anaesthetics will have on healing. Studies that measure the effect of EMLA on healing are required, although healing is not always the main priority for patients with chronic wounds. For some patients in the palliative care phase, symptom management becomes the priority.

References

Agrifoglio G, Domanin M, Baggio E, Cao, P, Alberti AN, Borin AR, et al (2000) EMLA anaesthetic cream for sharp debridement of venous leg ulcers: a double masked placebo controlled study. *Phlebology* 15(2): 81–3

American Geriatrics Society (1998) American Geriatrics Society. Panel on chronic pain in older persons. The management of chronic pain in older persons. *AGS* 46(5): 635–51

Aronoff GM, Brennan MJ, Pritchard DD, et al (2005) Evidence-based oral transmuscosal fentanyl citrate dosing guidelines. *Pain Med* 6(4): 305–14

Back IN, Finlay I (1995) The analgesic effect of topical opioids on painful skin ulcers. *J Pain Symptom Management* 10(7): 493

Ballantyne JC, Loach AB, Carr DB (1988) Itching after epidural and spinal opiates. *Pain* 33: 149–60

Ballas SK (2002) Treatment of painful sickle cell ulcers with topical opioids *Blood* 99(3): 1096

Bandolier (2008) NSAIDs and adverse effects 2008 [cited 0905/2008 2008]. Available online at: www.medicine.ox.ac.uk/bandolier/booth/painpag/nsae/nsae.html

Bush D, Bonney G (1992) Analgesia after surgery. *Br Med J* 305: 1160–1

Borland ML, Bergesio R, Pascoe EM, Turner S, Woodger S (2005) Intranasal fentanyl is an equivalent analgesic to oral morphine in paediatric burns patients for dressing changes: a randomised double blind crossover study. *Burns* 31(7): 831–7

Blanke and Hallern (2003) Sharp wound debridement in local anaesthesia using EMLA cream: 6 years experience in 1084 patients. *Eur J Emerg Med* 10(3): 229–31

Blower AL, Brooks A, Fenn CG (1997) Emergency admissions for upper gastrointestinal disease and their relation to NSAID use. *Aliment Pharmacol Ther* 11: 283–91

British National Formulary (2008) BNF 55. BMJ Group and RPS Publishing, London

Briggs M, Closs S (2006) Patients' perceptions of the impact of treatments and products on their experience of leg ulcer pain. *J Wound Care* 15: 333–7

Briggs M, Nelson EA (2003) Topical agents or dressings for pain in venous leg ulcers. Cochrane Database of Systematic Reviews Issue 1. Art. No.: CD001177. DOI: 10.1002/14651858.CD001177

Briggs M, Bennett MI, Cocks K, Closs SJ (2007) Painful leg ulceration: a prospective, longitudinal cohort study. *Wound Rep Regen* 15: 186–91

Briggs M, Flemming K (2007) Living with leg ulceration: a synthesis of qualitative research. _J Adv Nurs_ **59**: 319–28

British Pain Society (2004) Recommendations for the appropriate use of opioids for persistent non-cancer pain. British Pain Society, London. Available online at: www.britishpainsociety.org/book_opioid_main.pdf

Carr DB, Goudas LC (1999) Acute pain. _Lancet_ **353**: 2051–7

Coulling S (2007) Fundamentals of pain management in wound care. _Br J Nurs_ (Tissue Viability Supplement) **16**(11): S4–S12

Courade JP, Chassaing C, Bardin L (2001) 5-HT receptor subtypes involved in the spinal antinociceptive effect of acetaminophen in rats. _Eur J Pharmacol_ **432**: 1–7

Domenech RPI, Romanelli M, Tsiftsis DD, Slonkova V, Jortikka A, _et al_ (2008) Effect of an ibuprofen-releasing foam dressing on wound pain a real life. _J Wound Care_ **17**(8): 342–8

Edwards LM (2003) Why patients do not comply with compression bandaging. _Br J Nurs_ (Tissue Viability Supplement) **12**(11): S5–S16

Enander M, Domanin M, Baggio E, Cao P, Alberti AN, Borin AR, _et al_ (2000) EMLA anaesthetic cream for sharp debridement of venous leg ulcers: a double masked placebo controlled study. _Phlebology_ **15**(2): 81–3

Enander Malmros I, Nilsen T, Lillieborg S (1990) Plasma concentrations and analgesic effect of EMLA (Lidocaine/Prilocaine) cream for the cleansing of leg ulcers. _Acta Derm Venereol_ (Stockh)**70**: 227–30

Flanagan M, Vogensen H, Hasse L (2006) Case series investigating the experience of pain in patients with chronic venous leg ulcers treated with a foam dressing releasing ibuprofen. World Wide Wounds April Version 1 Last updated April 2006. Available online at: www.worldwidewounds.com

Flock P, Gibbs L, Sykes N (2000) Diamorphine-metronidazole gel effective for the treatment of painful infected ulcers. _J Pain Symptom Management_ **20**(6): 396–7

Flock P (2003) Pilot study to determine the effectiveness of diamorphine gel to control pressure ulcer pain. _J Pain Symptom Management_ **25**(6): 547–54

Gloth MF (1996) Concerns with chronic analgesic therapy in elderly patients. _Am J Med_ **101**(1A): 19–24

Gloth MF (2001) Pain management in older adults: Prevention and treatment. _Am Geriatr Soc_ **49**(2): 188–99

Goucke RC, Graziotti PJ (2003) Oral opioids and chronic non-cancer pain. In: Rice ASC, Warfield CA, Justins D, Eccleston C, eds. _Clinical Pain Management, Chronic Pain._ Arnold, London

Guarnera G, Tinelli G, Abeni D, Di Pietro C, Sampogna F, Tabolli S (2007)

Pain and quality of life in patients with vascular leg ulcers: an italian multicentre study. *J Wound Care* 16(8): 347–51

Gatchel RJ, Peng YB, Peters ML, Fuchs PN, Turk DC (2007) The biopsychosocial approach to chronic pain: scientific advances and future directions. *Psychological Bull* 133(4): 581–624

Gottrup F, Jorgensen B, Karlsmark T, *et al* (2007) Less pain with Biatain Ibu: initial findings from a randomised controlled double blind clinical investigation on painful venous leg ulcers. *Int Wound J* 4(suppl 1): 24–34

Hansson C, Holm J, Lillieborg S (1993) Repeated treatment with lidocaine/ prilocaine cream (EMLA) as a topical anaesthetic for the cleansing of venous ulcers: a controlled study. *Acta Derm Venereol* (Stockh) 73: 231–3

Haythornthwaite JA, Menefee LA, Quantro-Piacentini AL, Pappagallo M (1998) Outcome of chronic opioid therapy for non-cancer pain. *J Pain Symptom Management* 15(3): 185–94

Heffernan AM, Rowbotham DJ (2003) Clinical pharmacology: opioids. In: Rice ASC, Warfield CA, Justins D, Eccleston C, eds. *Clinical Pain Management, Acute Pain*. Arnold, London

Heinen MH, Person A, Van de Kerhof P, Otero M, Achterberg T (2007) Ulcer-related problems and health care needs in patients with venous leg ulceration: A descriptive, cross-sectional study. *Int J Nurs Stud* 44: 1296–1303

Helme RD, Katz B (2003) Chronic Pain in the Elderly. In: Jensen TS, Wilson PR, Rice ASC, eds. *Clinical Pain Management, Chronic Pain*. Arnold, London

Hersh EV (2000) Over the counter analgesics and antipyretics: a critical assessment. *Clin Ther* 22: 500–48

Hew de Laat E, Reimer W, Achterberg T (2005) Pressure ulcers: diagnostics and interventions aimed at wound-related complaints: a review of the literature. *J Clin Nurs* 14: 464–72

Holm J, Andren B, Grafford K (1990) EMLA vs placebo. *Acta Dermatologica Venereologica* 70: 132–6

Holst RG, Kristofferson A (1998) Lidocaine-prilocaine cream (EMLA cream) as a topical anaesthetic for the cleansing of leg ulcers. The effect of length of application time. *Eur J Dermatol* 8: 245–7

Hofman D (2006) Practical steps to address pain in wound care. *Br J Community Nurs Supplement* 15(1): 10–14

Johnson C, Repper J (1992) A double blind placebo controlled study of lidocaine/prilocaine cream (EMLA 5%) used as a topical analgesic for cleansing and redressing of leg ulcers. Confidential report from Astra Zeneca Pain Control AB

Jorgensen B, Frii GJ, Gottrup F (2006) Pain and quality of life for patients with venous leg ulcers: proof of concept of the efficacy of Biatain-Ibu, a new pain reducing wound dressing. *Wound Rep Regen* 14: 233–9

Krajnik M, Zylicz Z, Finlay I (1999) Potential uses of topical opioids in palliative care report of 6 cases. *Pain* 80: 121–5

Labate A, Newton MR, Vernon GM, Berkovic SF (2005) Tramadol and new-onset seizures. *Med J Aust* 182: 42–3

Layton AM, Ibbotson SH, Davies JA (1994) Randomised trial of oral aspirin for chronic venous leg ulcers. *Lancet* 344(3916): 164–5

Lok C, Paul C, Amblard P, Bessis D, Debure C, Faivre B, *et al* (1999) EMLA cream as a topical anaesthetic for the repeated mechanical debridement of venous leg ulcers: a double blind, placebo controlled study. *J Am Acad Dermatol* 40: 208–13

Macintyre PE, Jarvis DA (1996) Age is the best predictor of postoperative morphine requirement. *Pain* 64: 357–64

Macintyre PE, Upton RU, Ludbrook GL (2003) Acute pain management in the elderly patient. In: Rice ASC, Warfield CA, Justins D, Eccleston C, eds. *Clinical Pain Management Acute Pain*. Arnold, London

Mallett L (1999) Controlling the pain of venous leg ulceration. *Professional Nurse* 15: 131–4

Manning DC, Richer B(2003) Clinical pharmacology: non steroidal anti-inflammatory drugs. In: Rice ASC, Warfield CA, Justins D, Eccleston C, eds. *Clinical Pain Management Acute Pain*. Arnold, London

Maxwell T (2000) Cancer pain management in the elderly. *Geriatr Nurs* 21(3): 158–63

McGuire LK, Heffner R, Glaser B, Needleman W, Malarkey S, Dickinson S, *et al* (2006) Pain and wound healing in surgical patients. *Ann Behav Med* 31(2): 165–72

McQuay HJ (1999) Opioids in pain management. *Lancet* 353: 2229–32

Moore A, Collins S, Carroll D, McQuay H (1997) Paracetomol with and without codeine in acute pain: a quantitative systematic review. *Pain* 70: 193–201

Muth-Selbach US, Tegeder I, Brune K, Geisslinger G (1999) Acetaminophen inhibits spinal prostaglandin E2 release after peripheral noxious stimulation. *Anesthesiology* 91: 231–9

Moffatt C, Franks PJ, Hollinworth H (2002) Understanding wound pain and trauma: an international perspective. In: European Wound Management Association Position Document: *Pain at wound dressing changes*. London: MEP Ltd: 2–7

Pal SK, Cortiella J, Herndon D (1997) Adjunctive methods of pain control in burns. *Burns* 23(5): 404–12

Persoon A, Heinen MM, van der Vleuten CJ, *et al* (2004) Leg ulcers: a review of their impact on daily life. *J Clin Nurs* 13(3): 341–54

Poonawala T, Levay-Young BK, Hebbel RP, Gupta K (2005) Opioids heal ischemic wounds in the rat. *Wound Rep Regen* 13(2): 165–74

Ribeiro MDC, Zeppetella G (2002) Fentanyl for chronic pain. (Protocol) Cochrane Database of Systematic Reviews, Issue 1. Art. No: CD004235

Rice ASC, Maton S (2001.) Gabapentin in postherpetic neuralgia: a randomised, double blind, placebo controlled study. *Pain* 94: 215–24

Rosenthal D, Murphy F, Gottschalk R, Baxter M, Lycka B, Nevin K (2001) Using a topical anaesthetic cream to reduce pain during sharp debridment of chronic leg ulcers. *J Wound Care* 10(1): 503–5

Ruoff G (1998) The impact of nonsteroidal anti-inflammatory drugs on hypertension: alternative analgesics for patients at risk. *Clin Ther* 20(3): 376–87

Saarto T, Wiffen PJ (2007) Antidepressants for neuropathic pain. Cochrane Database of Systematic Reviews, Issue 4. Art. No: CD005454

Sibbald RG, Coutts P, Fierheller M (2006) Decreased chronic (persistent) wound pain with a novel sustained release ibuprofen foam dressing. Poster presented at European Wound Management Association, Prague, Czech Republic

Snaith ML (1992) Any questions? *Br Med J* 305: 812

Stein C (1995) Morphine — A local analgesic. *Int Assoc Study Pain Clinical Updates* 3(1): 1–8

Szor JK,d Bourguignon C (1999) Description of pressure ulcer pain at rest and at dressing change. *J Wound Ostomy Continence Nurs* 26: 115–20

Twillman RK (1999) Treatment of painful skin ulcers with topical opioids. *J Pain Symptom Management* 17(4): 289–92

Vanscheidt W, Lillieborg S (2001) EMLA anaesthetic cream for sharp debridement: a review of the clinical evidence for analgesic efficacy and tolerability. *Eur J Dermatol* 11(2): 90–6

Westerling D, Hoglund P, Lundin S, *et al* (1994) Transdermal administration of morpine to healthy subjects. *Br J Clin Pharmcol* 37: 571–6

World Health Organization (2008) Pain Relief and Palliative Care. WHO, Geneva. Available online at: www.who.int.

Wiffen PJ, McQuay HJ, Edwards JE, Moore RA (2005) Gabapentin for acute and chronic pain. Cochrane Database of Systematic Reviews, Issue 3. Art. No: CD005452. DOI: 10.1002/14651858.CD005452

Woo K, Sibbald G, Fogh K, Glynn C, Krasner D, Leaper D, *et al* (2008) Assessment and management of persistent chronic and total wound pain. *Int Wound J* 5(2): 205–11

Vermeire A, Remon JP (1999) Stability and compatibility of morphine. *Int J*

Pharm **87**: 17–51

Vernassiere C, Cornet C, Trechot P, Alla F, Truchetet F, Cuny JF, *et al* (2005) Study to determine the efficacy of topical morphine on painful chronic skin ulcers. *J Wound Care* **14**(6): 289–93

Zenz M, Strumpf M, Tyrba M (1992) Long term oral opioid therapy in patients with chronic non-malignant pain. *J Pain Symptom Management* **7**(2): 69–77

Zeppetella G (2001) Sublingual fentanyl citrate for cancer-related breakthrough pain: a pilot study. *Palliative Med* **15**: 323–8

CHAPTER 9

NON-PHARMACOLOGICAL METHODS OF PAIN CONTROL

Sabu James

There has been a growing body of evidence about the significant negative impact of chronic wound pain on the quality of life of patients (Franks *et al*, 1994; Price and Harding, 1996; Shukla *et al*, 2008). Adequate pain control is an important aspect of wound care management.

Underlying persistent pain, present even when the wound is not being manipulated, is what Krasner described (2001) in her model of chronic wound pain as, 'a cyclic acute pain'. This pain is associated with dressing changes. 'Non-cyclic acute' wound pain occurs during intermittent manipulation of the wound (Krasner, 2001), such as patient positioning, mobilisation, physiotherapy and occupational therapy. Such pain is understandably distressing for patients, especially children, and often the parent or carer feel helpless and upset themselves. One of the key issues for chronic wounds is that the dressing needs to be changed frequently, the wound has to be assessed, washed and medication applied. Pain is thus an inevitable part of wound care (Reid, 1996; Price, 1998; Neil and Munjas, 2000). A UK survey found that nurses considered preventing wound pain at dressing changes a challenging priority (Hollinworth, 1997; Hollinworth and Collier, 2000).

The distress that is caused can reduce compliance with wound management and impact adversely on healing, and in children can lead to complex behavioural issues (Hollinworth, 1997). Patients tend to dread wound dressing changes, cope poorly with mobilising and physiotherapy, which, in turn, can delay wound healing. Together with the varying degrees of disfigurement and malodour, this can lead to patients becoming depressed and socially isolated (Franks *et al*, 1994; Jones, 2008).

Why do wounds become painful?

Unless associated with sensory neuropathy, a chronic, non-healing wound is painful. Multi-drug resistant infections, vascular insufficiency, as well as malnutrition, poorly controlled diabetes (Caputo *et al*, 1997; Papanas and Edmonds, 2005), chemotherapy and radiotherapy can all contribute to poor healing, leading to chronicity of wounds. Smoking and other circulatory disorders can precipitate slow/inadequate wound healing and cause persisting pain. Extensive burns and resulting contractures result in severe pain and chronicity of wounds (*Chapter 7*).

The issue of pain is often overlooked in chronic wounds, as there is an assumption that the patient no longer feels pain when the dermis is destroyed together with the dermal nerve endings. However, the fact that patients with chronic leg ulceration talk about pain as being continuous and unrelenting refutes this assumption (Moffatt and Franks 2002). Pain may be related to soft tissue oedema which accompanies a chronic wound. This oedema can cause compression of tissues and affect structures or organs near the wound.

Some patients may become 'used to' a degree of pain and therefore feel that they should not mention it to healthcare professionals.

The key to assessing pain in patients with chronic wounds is to ask the patient, score the pain on a pain chart and look for signs of pain during dressing changes, when mobilising, and in the patient's day-to-day routine.

Monitoring patients' pain levels can also help to detect changes in the wound status, such as the presence or absence of infection. If infection is present, the bacteria and release of histamine in the wound area leads to tissue oedema, increased exudate and increased pain levels for the patient.

How does pain become chronic?

Any pain which persists for more than three months is defined as chronic pain. Development of chronic pain involves multiple interactions between the the peripheral nervous system (PNS), spinal cord and the brain. Changes in pain receptors and their threshold can happen both at peripheral and central level, which can persist for a long time, leading to chronicity of pain. Intense pain during various manipulations to the wound, i.e. physiotherapy, can cause spinal 'wind-up' and 'central sensitisation', thus perpetuating the chronicity of pain.

Chronic wound pain is persistent pain, present even when the wound is not being manipulated. The pain can be nociceptive, due to tissue injury, or neuropathic, due to nerve injury. On top of this are the other types of pain, for example, acute pain arising from dressing changes, pain associated with physiotherapy and wound debridement, and persisting background pain.

Why use non-pharmacological pain control?

Non-pharmacological methods are best used alongside other appropriate medications. Where conventional painkillers are having an adverse effect on the person, especially in cases of organ failure (renal, hepatic), or when minimal doses of painkillers are not tolerated due to their side-effects, non-pharmacological methods are advocated. Patients with burns experience excruciating pain during wound care, despite being on strong opioid medication, and so non-pharmaceutical methods have a role to play (Carrougher *et al*, 2003; Perry *et al*, 1981) (*Chapter 7*).

Rest pain is probably best controlled using the required dose of analgesics. However, during daily wound care procedures involving the removal of bandages, wound cleansing, assessment, disinfection and re-bandaging, opioid analgesics can often be inadequate as the intensity of the pain shoots up. This can lead to non-compliance with the therapy, especially in children with burn wounds who undergo repeated procedures (Blount *et al*, 1991). Excessive doses of opioids at this time, on top of the background dose, can cause increased side-effects, such as nausea and vomiting, sedation, and respiratory depression (Cherny *et al*, 2001) (*Chapter 8*). Educating patients about their expectations of pain and teaching them better coping strategies, along with pharmacological interventions, has been shown to be more effective than the latter on its own (Ferrell, 1996).

The following non-pharmacological methods of pain control can be considered alongside pharmacological interventions. The choice of one or more will depend on various factors such as age, gender, ethnicity and the choice of the patient, along with his/her carer/parent, as appropriate.

Acupuncture and acupressure

Acupuncture and acupressure have been used since ancient times in China and the Far East to manage pain, both acute and chronic. Historically, acupuncture is based on the belief that life forces or energy called 'Qi' (pronounced as Chi) move through the body along specific paths called 'meredians'. During acupuncture, a needle is inserted into the meredian that runs through the area of pain to interrupt it. It is believed that this stops, decreases or modifies the pain. Although the exact mechanism by which acupuncture works is a subject of debate, it is believed that endogenous opioids are released into the body. Recent studies support the idea of an enhanced production and release of nitric oxide which, in turn, improves local circulation (Ma, 2003; Tsuchiya _et al_, 2007). For those who have a phobia of needles, the conventional acupuncture needle can be substituted by laser acupuncture.

Anodyne therapy

This technique uses an array of infrared lights (Monochromatic infrared energy or MIRE), mounted on pads to gently warm the skin over a painful area. The heating effect is believed to release nitric oxide, improving circulation which, in turn, hastens the wound healing process (Inoue _et al_, 2003). The sight of a healing wound will also motivate patients to tolerate pain better (McCurdy, 2003). Anodyne therapy is used for managing chronic pain, especially as a result of diabetic neuropathy and microvascular insufficiency. Several studies have shown remarkable reduction in pain lasting for varying periods of time using this innovative technique (Leonard _et al_, 2004; Harkless _et al_, 2006).

Aromatherapy

Pleasant, familiar smells help aid relaxation, for example, scented candles and massage oils, can be used. Pleasant smells are believed to increase the production of endorphins. Besides creating a calming environment, aromatherapy also helps to mask the unpleasant odour of wounds.

Biofeedback

Although it takes a long time to master, biofeedback helps the body to respond differently to stressful situations, such as pain. It involves developing patients' ability to alter a particular physiological response by providing them with feedback about the response they are attempting to control. Relaxing more can help to lessen pain, thereby making it more tolerable. However, pain is viewed as a homeostatic emotion, constantly evolving with multimodal physical, physiological, psychological and pathological components, not merely a sensory experience (Craig, 2003). Biofeedback is most beneficial if used together with other techniques of pain control (Gatchel *et al*, 2003). In combination with cognitive behavioural therapy (CBT), it can increase a patient's sense of self-efficiency, providing clear feedback about his/her ability to gain control over certain physiological responses.

Breathing exercises and relaxation techniques

Gently breathing in and out, focusing on a distant sound or listening to soothing music can help a patient to relax (Carroll and Seers, 1998). Meditative breathing is another such technique (Van Fleet, 2000; Ryman and Rankin-Box, 2001). Meditative breathing has its roots in Buddhism and Yoga. One starts by finding a quiet place and getting comfortable, attention being given to breathing. Brief relaxation (where deep breathing is used to trigger relaxation throughout the body) and tension relaxation exercises (alternate tensing and relaxing of muscle groups) are other relaxation techniques that can be used.

Cognitive behavioural therapy (CBT)

CBT helps by changing the way we think and react to situations which are complex. It has been found to be useful in anxiety, depression, panic, and bulimia nervosa. CBT is also widely used as one of the psychological interventions for chronic pain management (Turner and Chapman, 1982). It is not an overnight process, but requires an expert therapist for success. The use of CBT has been extended to children and adolescents, and it is best when combined with biofeedback mechanisms (Hoffman, 2008).

Distraction therapy

Anticipation of pain can lead to an increased intensity in pain and subsequent discomfort. Diverting the patient's attention, especially while managing wound dressings in children, can have a significant effect on coping with pain (*Chapter 5*). Computerised virtual reality and computer games can help here. Although these may seem time-consuming and expensive, they have been shown to be effective in gaining patients' trust and improving comfort during procedures (Patterson *et al*, 1997; Peyron *et al*, 1999; Rainville *et al*, 1999; Hoffman *et al*, 2000) .

Environmental context

Some recent theories of pain highlight the role that external sensory stimuli can play in the pain experience (Melzack, 1999; Craig, 2003). Keefe *et al* (2008) have explored the influence of stimuli such as light, nature and sounds, as well as video and virtual reality (VR) on pain. Patients who were treated in rooms with brighter natural light experienced less pain, and required less pain medication. Serotonin levels may increase by exposure to light, which can impact on pain. Vitamin D levels also rise, which again may help to decrease pain (Keefe *et al*, 2008). Portable video or virtual reality (VR) kiosks could be made available in treatment facilities. However, repeated viewing of the same material decreases the positive effects (Miller *et al*, 1992) and so a variety of materials should be available.

Guided imagery

Conjuring up pleasant images in your brain can help to improve well-being. Imagining that you are in a less stressful situation helps to decrease the intensity of pain (Ryman and Rankin-Box, 2001; Van Fleet, 2000). This technique, as with others in this chapter, requires training from psychologists and other healthcare professionals.

Hypnosis

Hypnosis is not a treatment in itself, but a set of techniques designed to improve concentration, minimise distractions and heighten responsiveness to suggestions, thus altering one's thoughts, feelings, behaviour or physiological states. The effectiveness of hypnosis to decrease sensitivity to pain — known as hypno-analgesia — has been seen in well-controlled experiments, with pain relief being one of the most researched areas (Wakeman and Kaplan, 1978; Turner and Chapman, 1982; Patterson *et al*, 1992). The key to becoming hypnotised is the extent to which a person is hypnotisable. Since pain associated with chronic wounds is intense during interventions, such as dressing changes and cleansing, it can be considered an acute, short-living pain, for which hypnosis can be effective. Hypnosis can help to alleviate the sensory and/or affective components of the intense pain experience (Patterson *et al*, 1997; Peyron *et al*, 1999; Rainville *et al*, 1999; Hoffman *et al*, 2000).

Low level laser therapy (LLLT)

LLLT involves application of a non-thermal, multi-wave length laser to the wound surface. It has been shown to reduce pain when used as a palliative treatment for fungating wounds (Humzah *et al*, 1993).

Modelling

This technique is more applicable to children than adults. It has been used in studies of reducing needle-related distress (Duff *et al*, 2004). Modelling is based on the principle that watching another child (preferably of the same sex, age group and ethnicity) displaying some anxiety about needle insertion, but overcoming it, will help the observing child to utilise successful coping skills. This can also be done by watching video clips, CD-ROMS or even interactive computer games. This technique is also used to teach parents how to distract and interact with their child during venepuncture (Bauchner *et al*, 1994).

Music therapy

Singing, humming, listening to music or playing an instrument helps to release endorphins and increase cerebral circulation. Endorphins play an important role in the endogenous analgesic circuit, raising pain threshold and probably play a role in potentiating the descending inhibitory pain pathways/control. Improved cerebral circulation improves mood and increases energy levels (Richards *et al*, 2007). Patients with burns reported significant reduction in pain when listening to music, in contrast to those who did not receive music therapy (Fratianne _et al_, 2001). This can be combined with video recordings composed of scenic beauty or other music-based imagery (Miller _et al_, 1992).

Presence of parent/carer presence during procedure

The presence of a parent or carer during procedures such as dressing changes can calm patients, especially children. Familiar faces not only create strong bonds and trust, but the person gets to learn the pain threshold of the patient as well.

Snoezelon

This is described as a multi-sensory area with equipment to create a dynamic environment, offering stimulating input (auditory, visual, olfactory and tactile). This may help infants and pre-schoolers to become calm prior to, or following painful interventions. Here, experiences are arranged to stimulate primary senses, without the need for intellectual activity, thus facilitating relaxation (Duff and Bliss, 2005).

Transcutaneous electrical nerve stimulation (TENS)

TENS is believed to work on the 'gate control' mechanism in the spinal cord. It produces its effect by stimulating large diameter nerve fibres (Aβ-fibres) that carry signals to the spinal cord and inhibit transmission of pain signals (_Chapter 4_) (Rook, 1996; Hasson and Lundberg, 1999). TENS is also believed to be effective in relieving the itching that can be associated with fungating wounds (Grocott, 2000).

Transcutaneous spinal electroanalgesia (TSE)

TSE is similar to TENS but the pulses are of higher voltage and shorter duration (a few millionths of a second in duration). Since the pulse duration is extremely short, patients feel only a mild tingling sensation, unlike TENS, and the therapy is well tolerated (Macdonald and Coates, 1995). The pads have to be applied on either side of the neck for head and facial pain. For all other sources of pain, there are two pad positions — one on the spinous process of T1 (first thoracic vertebra) and the second on the T12 (spinous process of twelfth thoracic vertebra). An improvement in mood and tension has been reported in adults after application of TSE over the spine (Towell *et al*, 1997).

Touch therapy and massage

Gently massaging the back, shoulders, and neck can help a patient to relax, and this, together with music, breathing exercises and other forms of distraction, can help to lessen the intensity of pain. The patient along with his/her carer or a healthcare professional can practice these techniques so that they can be used effectively during painful procedures (Turner *et al*, 1998). The presence of regular carers, parents or a friendly face contribute significantly to managing pain in difficult situations, especially in patients with intellectual disabilities.

Virtual reality (VR) pain control

One of the first studies to test the efficacy of virtual reality as a means of pain control was Hoffman *et al* (2000). The greatest decreases in pain and anxiety were reported in patients who felt that they were in the VR environment. They repeated this study recently with partial immersion technique in water with VR, and the results showed less pain perception (Hoffman *et al*, 2008).

Summary and conclusion

Acute exacerbation of longstanding chronic pain associated with poorly healing or non-healing wounds can be effectively managed by using one or more of the interventions mentioned above, along with appropriate medication. Only some of the techniques may be suitable for children, e.g. virtual reality pain control techniques, music, snoezelon, distraction techniques, and presence of carer or parent. Many of the techniques like CBT, biofeedback and guided imagery will initially need trained healthcare professionals like psychologists and behavioural therapists. Subsequently, all members of the multidisciplinary team, as well as carers/parents, who are regularly involved in patient care, can be trained.

If used in conjunction with an adequate dose of pain-killers, a gradual increase in the effectiveness of the non-pharmacological methods and a decrease in the dose of drugs may be observed. Some techniques will be time-consuming and expensive, such as VR and anodyne therapy, but by helping to increase patient compliance they hasten wound healing. The clinical effectiveness of non-pharmacological techniques mentioned in the management of wound-related pain still requires further investigations (Carroll _et al_, 2001).

A recent study advocated new trials with strict research designs before revising current evidence-based recommendations. A study protocol comparing the effectiveness of acupuncture along with compression therapy and low-adherence dressings has been published and the results are awaited (Vas _et al_, 2008).

In conclusion, the right choice of analgesics, educating both patient and carer about anticipation of pain together with appropriate non-pharmacological intervention of pain control provides the best conditions for pain management of chronic wounds. It is important that wounds are assessed regularly and all therapeutic decisions discussed with patients, who should be involved throughout the process of wound pain management.

References

Barrett S (2007) 'Heal Not Hurt': piloting an initiative on wound pain assessment. _Br J Community Nurs_ 12: S18–S21

Bauchner H, Vinci R, May A (1994) Teaching parents how to comfort their children during common medical procedure. _Arch Dis Child_ 70: 548–50

Blount RL, Landolf-Fritsche B, Powers SW, Sturges JW (1991) Differences between high and low coping children and betwen parent and staff behaviors during painful procedures. _J Paediatr Psychol_ 16: 795–809

Caputo GM, Joshi N, Weitekamp MR (1997) Foot infections in patients with diabetes. _Am Family Physician_ 56(1): 195–202

Carroll D, Moore RA, McQuay HJ, Fairman F, Tramer M, Leijon G (2001) Transcutaneous electrical nerve stimulation (TENS) for chronic pain. _Cochrane Database Syst Rev_ 3: CD003222

Carroll D, Seers K (1998) Relaxation techniques for the relief of chronic pain: a systematic review. _J Adv Nurs_ 27: 476–87

Carrougher GJ, Ptacek JT, Sharar SR, _et al_ (2003) Comparison of patient satisfaction and self-reports of pain in adult burn-injured patients. *J Burn Care Rehabil* **24**: 1–8

Cherny N, Ripamonti C, Pereira J, *et al* (2001) Expert Working Group of the European Association of Palliative Care Network. Strategies to manage the adverse effects of oral morphine: an evidence-based report. *J Clin Oncol* **19**: 2542–54

Craig AD (2003) A new view of pain as a homeostatic emotion. *Trends Neurosci* **26**: 303–7

Duff AJA, Bliss AK (2005) Reducing distress during venupuncture. In: David TJ, ed. *Recent Advances in Paediatrics*. RSM Press, London: 149–65

Ferrell B (1996) Patient education and non-drug interventions. In: Ferrell BR, Ferrell BA, eds. *Pain in the Elderly*. IASP Press Seattle, WA

Franks PJ, Moffatt CJ, Oldroyd M, *et al* (1994) Community leg ulcer clinics: Effect on quality of life. *Phlebology* **9**(2): 83–6

Fratianne RB, Presner JD, Houston MJ, Super DM, Yowler CJ, Standley JM (2001) The effect of music-based imagery and musical alternate engagement on the burn debridement process. *J Burn Care Rehab* **22**(1): 47–53

Gatchel RJ, Robinson RC, Pulliam C, Maddrey AM (2003) Biofeedback with pain patients: Evidence for its effectiveness. *Semin Pain Med* **1**: 55–66

Grocott P (2000) Palliative management of fungating malignant wounds. *J Community Nurs* **14**(3): 31–8

Harkness LB, DeLellis S, Carnegie DH, Burke TJ (2006) Improved foot sensitivity and pain reduction in patients with peripheral neuropathy after treatment with Monochromatic Infra-red Energy (MIRE). *J Diabetes Complications* **20**(2): 81–7

Hasson P, Lundberg T (1999) Transcutaneous electrical nerve stimulation, vibration and acupuncture as pain relieving measures. In: Wall PD, Melzack R, eds. *Textbook of Pain*. 4th edn. Churchill Livingstone, Edinburgh

Hoffman HG, Patterson DR, Carrougher GJ (2000) Use of virtual reality for adjunctive treatment of adult burn pain during physical therapy: a controlled study. *Clin J Pain* **16**(3): 244–50

Hoffman HG, Patterson DR, Seibel E, Soltani M, Jewett-Leahy L, Sharar SR (2008) Virtual reality pain control during burn wound debridement in the hydrotank. *Clin J Pain* **24**(4): 299–304

Hollinworth H (1997) Less pain more gain. *Nurs Times* **93**(46): 89–91

Hollinworth H, Collier M (2000) Nurses' views about pain and trauma at dressing changes: results of a national survey. *J Wound Care* **9**(8): 369–73

Humzah MD, Diamantopoulas C, Dyson M (1993) Multi-wavelength low-reactive level laser therapy as an adjunct in malignant ulcers: case reports. *Laser Therapy* 5: 149–52

Inoue M, Sato EF, Nishikawa M, Park AM, Kira Y, Imada I, Utsumi K (2003) Cross talk of nitric oxide, oxygen radicals and super-oxide dismutase regulates the energy metabolism and cell death, and determines the fate of aerobic life. *Antioxid Redox Signal* 5: 475–84

Jones JE (2008) Impact of exudate and odour from chronic venous leg ulceration. *Nurs Standard* 22(45): 53–61

Keefe FJ, Malenbaum S, Williams AC de C, Ulrich R, Somers TJ (2008) Pain in its environmental context: Implications for designing environments to enhance pain control. *Pain* 134(3): 241–4

Krasner D (2001) Caring for the person experiencing chronic wound pain. In: Krasner DL, Rodeheaver GT, Sibbald RG, eds. *Chronic Wound Care: A Clinical Source Book for Healthcare Professionals*. 3rd ed. Wayne, PA: HMP Publications

Leonard DR, Farooqi MH, Myers S (2004) Restoration of sensation, reduced pain and improved balance in subjects with diabetic peripheral neuropathy. *Diabetes Care* 27(1): 168–72

Ma SX (2003) Enhanced nitric oxide concentrations and expression of nitric oxide synthase in acupuncture points/meridians. *J Altern Complement Med* 9: 207–15

Macdonald AJR, Coates TW (1995) The discovery of transcutaneous spinal electro analgesia and its relief of chronic pain. *Physiotherapy* 81(11): 653–61

Malenbaum S, Keefe FJ, Williams AC, Ulrich R, Somers TJ (2008) Pain in its environmental context: implications for designing environments to enhance pain control. *Pain* 134(3): 241–4. Epub 2008 Jan 4

McCurdy B (2003) Technology in Practice: Is anodyne therapy the answer for peripheral neuropathy? *Podiatry Today* 16(4): 78–80

Melzack R (1999) From the gate to the neuromatrix. *Pain* 6: S121–6

Miller AC, Hickmann LC, Lemasters GK (1992) A distraction technique for control of burn pain. *J Burn Care Rehabil* 13: 576–80

Neil JA, Munjas BA (2000) Living with a chronic wound: the voice of sufferers. *Ostomy Wound Management* 46(5): 28–38

Papanas N, Edmonds N (2005) Facing the real necessities in the diabetic foot. *Diabetic Foot* 8(3): 118–19

Patterson DR, Adcock RJ, Bombardier CH (1997) Factors predicting hypnotic analgesia in clinical burn pain. *Int J Clin Exp Hypn* 45(4): 377–95

Perry S, Heidrich G, Ramos E (1981) Assessment of pain by burn patients. *J Burn Care Rehabil* 2: 322–7

Peyron R, García-Larrea L, Grégoire MC, *et al* (1999) Hemodynamic brain responses to acute pain in humans: sensory and attentional networks. *Brain* **122**(Pt 9): 1765–80

Price P, Harding KG (1996) Measuring health-related quality of life in patients with chronic leg ulcers. *WOUNDS* **8**(3): 91–94

Price P (1998) Health-related quality of life and the patient's perspective. *J Wound Care* **7**(7): 365–6

Rainville P, Hofbauer RK, Paus T, Duncan GH, Bushnell MC, Price DD (1999) Cerebral mechanisms of hypnotic induction and suggestion. *J Cogn Neurosci* **11**(1): 110–25

Reid J (1996) Quality of life measurement tool: using appropriate scales. *J Wound Care* **5**(3): 142

Richards T, Johnson J, Sparks A, Emerson H (2007) The effect of music therapy on patients' perception and manifestation of pain, anxiety and patient satisfaction. *Med Surg Nurs* **16**: 7–14

Rook JL (1996) Wound care pain management. *Adv Wound Care* **9**(6): 24–31

Ryman L, Rankin-Box D (2001) Relaxation and visualization. In: Rankin-Box, ed. *The Nurse's Handbook of Complementary Therapies*. 2nd edn. WB Saunders, London: 251–8

Shukla VK, Shukla D, Tripathi AK, Agrawal S, Tiwary SK, Prakash V (2008) Results of a one-day, descriptive study of quality of life in patients with chronic wounds. *Ostomy Wound Management* **54**(5): 43–9

Towell AD, William D, Boyd SG (1997) High frequency, non-invasive stimulation over the spine: effects on mood and mechanical pain tolerance in normal subjects. *Behav Neurol* **10**: 61–5

Tsuchiya M, Sato EF, Inoue M, Asada A (2007) Acupuncture enhances generation of nitric oxide and increases local circulation. *Anesth Analg* **104**: 301–7

Turner JA, Chapman CR (1982) Psychological interventions for chronic pain: A critical review: II. Operant conditioning, hypnosis and cognitive behavior therapy. *Pain* **12**: 23–46

Turner JG, Clark AJ, Gauthier DK, Williams M (1998) The effect of therapeutic touch on pain and anxiety in burn patients. *J Adv Nurs* **28**: 10–20

Van Fleet S (2000) Relaxation and imagery for symptom management: improving patient assessment and individualising treatment. *Oncol Nurs Forum* **27**(3): 501–10

Vas J, Modesto M, Mendez C, *et al* (2008) Effectiveness of acupuncture, special dressings and simple, low-adherence dressings for healing venous leg ulcers in primary healthcare: study protocol for a cluster-randomized open-labelled trial. *BMC Complement Altern Med* **8**: 29

Chapter 10

Patient-controlled Analgesia

Kath Clarke and Ron Iphofen

Pain is a sensation experienced by all human beings, its nature depending upon a range of influences including causal factors (Carr and Mann, 2000, *p. 2*), intensity (MacLellan, 2006, *p. 3*), personal experience (Moore *et al*, 2003, *p. 7*), mood (Sofaer and Walker, 1994) and cultural beliefs (MacLellan, 2006, *p. 65*). Defining pain is notoriously difficult, but the current consensus draws on the International Association for the Study of Pain (IASP) which defines pain as an unpleasant sensory and emotional experience associated with actual or potential tissue damage, or described in terms of such damage (IASP, 1994, 1979). This definition attempts to consider the multi-dimensional aspects of the pain experience, including the psychological factors that can influence the experience, as well as delineating a phenomenon, which everyone has experienced, but which people frequently struggle to describe. Due to the subjective nature of pain, its management poses difficulties for the healthcare professional. One patient's pain cannot be compared to another, even if the source of the pain comes from a similar incident, for example, post-operative pain after abdominal surgery. Consequently, individualising post-operative pain treatment is the key to improved pain management (Macintyre and Ready, 1996, *p. 54*).

Disease, injury and surgical procedures are associated with pain in varying degrees. Nurses, whether in primary or secondary care, will provide pain assessment, management and advice to patients on a daily basis. During the 1980s, patient-controlled analgesia (PCA) was introduced into acute pain management, allowing patients to titrate their own analgesic requirement, thus improving patient satisfaction and heralding a breakthrough in post-operative pain management (Carter Snell *et al*, 1997). Patients self-administering oral analgesia is an example of patient-controlled analgesia in its simplest form. Today, PCA is commonly used after surgery, although it has a role in the management of trauma pain, incident or procedural pain, and pre-operative pain when a patient is unable to take anything orally. PCA is appropriate for use in the management of wound pain in the acute surgical setting and can be seen as the treatment of choice within acute hospitals. The use of intravenous PCA is limited within the community because of the level of monitoring required for this type of treatment.

Lehman (2005) sees PCA as being based on the principle of WYNIWYG (what you need is what you get). This allows the patient to titrate their analgesia requirement according to the pain they are experiencing. It empowers the patient and allows them to take control of their pain without recourse to the nursing or medical staff. As the patient achieves pain control through titrating only the amount of the drug they require, there is less likelihood of side-effects such as sedation and nausea (Thomas, 1997, *p. 166*).

PCA can be provided via various routes using different agents to deliver the desired outcome of controlled pain (*Table 10.1*). The principles, however, remain the same.

PCA infusion pumps and devices

Today, there are various infusion pumps and devices on the market that can deliver analgesia in a controlled and on-demand manner.

Table 10.1: Routes to deliver pain control		
Route	Agent	Background infusion (with/without)
Intravenous	• Morphine • Pethidine • Fentanyl	+/- +/- -
Epidural	• Fentanyl and bupivacaine • Bupivacaine • Ropivacaine	+/- +/- +/-
Intrapleural regional block	• Bupivacaine • Ropivacaine	- -
Intranasal	• Diamorphine	-
Inhalation	• Entonox	-

The pump needs to have the following facilities to enable a patient to administer their own analgesia:

- *Concentration:* this is the concentration of the drug being used, e.g. morphine 1 mg/ml or pethidine 10 mg/ml.
- *PCA bolus dose:* the amount of analgesia that will be delivered on each successful patient demand.
- *Lockout interval:* the period of time that has to elapse before the pump will deliver another dose on patient demand, ensuring that the dose administered has time to exert its full analgesic effect.
- *Loading dose:* this is a dose that is programmed as a once-only dose and is usually given when treatment starts, occasionally it can be used prior to a painful procedure, such as dressing change.
- *Background infusion (if required):* a background infusion is a continuous infusion that runs in conjunction with PCA. It is usually used when the patient is in an area of close patient monitoring, such as a high dependency unit, as the patient is more at risk of sedation and respiratory depression.

The pump is programmed to provide a specific amount of analgesia on patient demand, usually when a button is pressed, with the pump 'locking out' for a specified set time period to ensure that the patient cannot have too much of the drug. A maximum dose of the analgesic that can be delivered in a set time period may also be programmed. A loading dose is usually given at the start of treatment when the PCA is initiated to obtain control of acute pain in a short period of time. Within the context of wound care, a loading dose might be given prior to a wound being debrided or additionally during the debridement should the patient's pain require it. A dedicated intravenous line connects the pump to the patient, this serves to maintain the patency of the line, particularly when PCA is only being used occasionally. This line also has an anti-siphon valve which prevents the analgesic solution backing up the Y connector if the cannula should become occluded, thereby preventing undesired, large amounts of the analgesic being delivered once an occluded line is cleared. Once this initial pain control has been achieved, it becomes practical to hand over the control to the patient for continued self-administration, rather than clinician-administration.

Suggested regimens for the various routes of PCA in adults are illustrated in *Table 10.2* and, although care has been taken to ensure that drug selections and dosages are in accordance with currently accepted practice, it is recommended that all suggested regimens are reviewed in the light of current practice.

Some of the PCA infusion pumps on the market have a facility that allows a history of events to be downloaded, although a visual history readout should be available for safety reasons.

The principles of intravenous PCA can be applied to other routes such as epidural, regional blocks, intranasal or inhalation. Epidural infusions have the additional benefit of patient-controlled epidural analgesia (PCEA), which allows the patient to deliver on demand an additional 'top-up' dose of analgesia via the epidural route. This is particularly useful as an additional loading dose prior to a painful procedure, such as a dressing change, removal of a drain or

Table 10.2: Suggested PCA regimens for adults (intranasal for paediatric use)

Route	Drug	Loading dose	PCA dose	Lockout interval	Background infusion
Intravenous	Morphine	0–10 mg	1 mg	5 minutes	Based upon patient's opiate naivity and need
	Pethidine	0–100 mg	10 mg	10 minutes	
	Fentanyl	0–100 mcg	10 mcg	5 minutes	Nil
Epidural	Bupivacaine 0.5% (5 mg/ml)	up to 20 mls	2–5 mls	15–30 minutes	0–20 mls
	Fentanyl 2 mcg per ml and bupivacaine 0.1%	Up to 20 mls	2–5 mls	15–30 minutes	0–15 mls
Regional nerve blocks: intrapleural	Bupivacaine 0.25% plus adrenaline 1:200 000	Up to 20 mls	9 mls	60 minutes	Nil
Intrathecal	Available but refer to specialised pain teams for advice and mangement				
Inhalation	Entonox	Nil	According to the inhaled breath	As the patient wishes to take	Nil
Intranasal (paediatric use)	Diamorphine 0.1 mg per kilo of child's weight, made up to the required volume to deliver the dose in 0.2 mls of sodium chloride 0.9%	Nil	0.2 mls	Single dose only	Nil

physiotherapy. Regional nerve blocks, such as intrapleural analgesia used following cholecystectomy or trauma resulting in fractured ribs, can use a PCA facility to allow the patient to provide pain relief on top of a continuous infusion (Clarke, 1999). Devices are available to facilitate other modes of delivery, such as disposable atomisers for intranasal PCA. These deliver a small volume of drug as programmed and are particularly useful for children in the accident and emergency department when venous access is difficult and pain relief is needed quickly (McDonald and Cooper, 2001; Shelley and Paech, 2008; Viscusi, 2008). Entonox$^{®}$ has similar advantages, as it can be administered quickly without venous access. Entonox is a mix of gases (50% oxygen and 50% nitrous oxide) and is supplied in pre-mixed cylinders. The mixture is inhaled by the patient using a demand valve attached to a face mask. It is particularly known for its use in labour pain (Bhattacharya *et al*, 2006), although it already has a use in incident pain (Evans, 2003).

Efficacy and safety of PCA

There is much literature which explores the efficacy and safety of PCA (Sidebotham and Schug, 1997; Walder *et al*, 2001; Lehman, 2005), as well as considering the nursing time saved through not having to prepare intramuscular injections (Koh and Thomas, 1994) and improved patient satisfaction (Carter Snell *et al*, 1997). PCA is considered to be the gold standard of acute pain management and its continuous developments in: pump delivery improvements; choice of analgesia; management of side-effects; and choice of route has maintained this standard. Nursing staff and patients alike are familiar with the concept and patients are reassured to know that major surgery will be followed by pain management using the PCA technique (Carter Snell *et al*, 1997).

Thomas and Rose (1993) identified three important factors for the optimum method of analgesic administration:

- mechanism of action of analgesics
- individual response of patients to the analgesic
- the subjectivity of the pain experience.

PCA recognises these three factors and, through the patient-controlled feature, it allows patients to administer the minimum effective analgesia needed for pain relief. The flexibility of the PCA regimen, which provides the patient with small and frequent bolus doses of opioid given as often as needed, is more likely to maintain a reasonably constant blood concentration of the drug; a concentration that, ideally, is kept within the analgesic 'corridor' for each patient (Macintyre and Ready, 1996, *p. 76*). However, as said, to obtain initial pain relief, on starting PCA the patient is given a loading dose so that blood levels rapidly reach the minimum effective analgesia concentration (MEAC), before control is given back to the patient to allow for the individualisation of the subjective experience.

The surgical nurse's role in PCA

The role of the nurse in PCA can be broken down into four stages:

1. Believing the patient with pain
2. Assessment
3. Education
4. Monitoring.

Believing the patient with pain

Any pain assessment must begin with believing the patient reporting the pain (Waterhouse, 1996), and successful pain management is dependent upon accurate pain assessment (Plaisance and Logan, 2006). Although this is obvious, it is the perception of being disbelieved by healthcare professionals that patients with acute and chronic pain complain about most often (Seers and Friedli, 1996; Clarke and Iphofen, 2005). Studies exploring the experience of living with pain frequently cite this feeling of being disbelieved as contributing to the overwhelming sense of despair and helplessness associated with chronic pain (Smith and Friedemann, 1999; Clarke and Iphofen, 2008). Any doubt on the part of the healthcare professional as to the extent of the pain that the patient is suffering usually results in poor analgesia through under-medication (Salmon and Manyande, 1996). Providing a patient with PCA empowers them to control their own pain, and, although studies have shown that opiate requirements are comparable with other methods, it does appear to improve patient satisfaction (Walder *et al*, 2001).

Assessment

PCA is no longer a new concept and the majority of surgical nurses will be familiar with the principle, although PCA is not suitable for every patient. The nurse will have to assess the patient's pain as well as their suitability for PCA. PCA relies on a patient pressing a button to enable the pump to deliver the analgesia, and the patient has to understand and feel safe with the concept as well as having the physical ability to press the demand button. Suitability for post-operative PCA should, where possible, be decided prior to surgery. The patient should have been given adequate information to ensure that they are aware of their role in post-operative pain management. Poor explanation will lead to poorly managed pain (Shade, 1992).

There are various tools available to aid the nurse in assessing a patient's pain (Platt and Byrnes, 2006; Bruckenthal and D'Arcy, 2007; Hall, 2007), although in the acute post-operative period a simple and quick form of assessment is appropriate, as this is not an ideal time to attempt a lengthy pain assessment.It is sufficient to ascertain whether the patient has pain and whether it is mild, moderate or severe and treat accordingly (Figure *10.1*). Pain assessment should be tailored to the patient and situation, and at the time of a wound dressing changes should be more detailed, particularly if the wound is chronic and the pain is persistent with acute exacerbation (World Union of Wound Healing Societies [WUWHS], 2007).

Education

It is equally important to educate both the patients and staff. Patients and their relatives should understand the concept of PCA. It is important that PCA remains in the control of the patient and that relatives do not press the demand button on their behalf, as this may mean that the patient is being given an analgesic dose when it is not required, increasing the risk of unwanted side-effects. Patient education must include clear explanations of the benefits as well as the potential side-effects of PCA. Written patient information should be provided. The patient also needs to be able to operate the demand button and nursing staff should check that they can reach the handset, particularly following surgery. Patients are encouraged to keep themselves comfortable with PCA, although some patients will aim to be 'pain-free'. It is difficult to keep a patient completely pain-

Assessment	0	1	2	3
Pain	No pain	Mild pain	Moderate pain	Severe pain
Nausea and vomiting	No nausea or vomiting	Nausea	Experiencing nausea with some vomiting	Severe vomiting
Sedation	Awake	Drowsy	Sleeping but possible to awaken	Unrousable

Figure 10.1: Scoring system to assess pain

free following surgery (unless epidural analgesia is being used), and explanation needs to be given to the patient that the aim of PCA is to keep them comfortable to minimise post-operative complications, such as deep vein thrombosis (DVT) or chest infection. PCA should provide enough comfort from pain to enable the patient to do their physiotherapy exercises and to take regular deep breaths.

All medical and nursing staff who initiate PCA must be familiar with the programming of the pump, its functions and the principles of caring for patients receiving PCA. It should only be initiated by nurses who have been assessed as being competent to do so. Competencies will cover programming of the pump, care of the patient using PCA, knowledge of the drugs being used, recognition and management of the side-effects of PCA and the monitoring of the patient, and how to change the syringe or infusion bag once empty.

Monitoring

The sole purpose for the monitoring of patients receiving PCA is to ensure the patient's safety. Any form of monitoring is to identify the early signs of side-effects and to prompt the nurse to take action appropriately. Individual hospitals will have their own monitoring charts for PCA, which are usually used in conjunction with vital sign observation charts. Assessment and monitoring of pain, sedation and nausea should be continued throughout the period that PCA is used. Simple assessment tools are effective and provide the nurse with enough information to ensure that the patient is comfortable. Within the acute post-operative setting a simple 0–3 scoring system can be used (*Figure 10.1*).

Side-effects from PCA

Side-effects are associated with opiates, rather than the concept of PCA itself. However, inadequate pain control could be seen as a possible side-effect if it is as a result of the patient not fully understanding the PCA concept, further demonstrating the importance of clear explanations.

Nausea and vomiting

Opioids do have some potential nausea and vomiting side-effects, which are often minimised by the use of PCA with the patient only receiving the amount of opiate needed to control the pain. A regular antiemetic should be prescribed and administered if the patient experiences nausea and vomiting. Some hospital PCA regimes combine an antiemetic with the analgesia (Kontrimaviciute _et al_, 2005; Boonmak _et al_, 2007). Not all patients experience nausea and vomiting and the ethical question thus arises as to whether the patient should be given a drug that is not required. Also, sometimes the surgery itself causes nausea and vomiting and so the fault may not entirely be with the opiate.

Sedation

Opiates may cause drowsiness and regular monitoring of the level of sedation is an essential component of patient monitoring. Most patients following surgery will experience a level of post-surgery fatigue and sleeping is not a problem, providing the patient is able to maintain hydration, nutrition and compliance with physiotherapy regimens and deep breathing exercises. Sleeping, however, can lead to an increase in pain as the patient is unable to press the demand button while asleep. The patient should be aware that, on waking, to get back on top of the pain, the demand button needs to be pressed every five minutes until pain control has been achieved. In some instances, a rescue PCA dose may be needed and this should be administered by a nurse with competency in this area, as a loading dose where prescribed.

Respiratory depression

Although there is no doubt that opioid analgesics can and do cause respiratory depression, this is usually a side-effect of larger doses (BNF, 2008, *p.* 229). The titration of analgesia according to the patient's individual pain experience ensures that respiratory depression is rarely seen as a consequence of PCA (Polomano *et al*, 2008), although if a continuous background infusion is in progress the risk of a respiratory depressive episode is increased (Sidebotham and Schug, 1997). As a matter of precaution, naloxone hydrochloride, a specific opioid antidote, should always be prescribed and made easily available.

Itching

Pruritus or itching is an uncomfortable side-effect that is often seen with opioids. Although this is not dangerous, it can be extremely unpleasant for the patient and so an antihistamine drug should be prescribed and administered regularly. Although Tarcatu *et al* (2007) describe how a small amount of intravenous naloxone was successful in relieving a patient's itching when traditional use of anti-histamines was not.

PCA in incident pain

Incident or procedural pain is defined as pain that is associated with a procedure such as physiotherapy or a dressing change (Macintyre and Ready, 1996, *p.* 78), although Kazanowski and Laccetti (2002, *p.* 77) state that incident pain could also be a reaction to emotional stimuli. One of the main advantages of a PCA regimen is that it provides the flexibility needed to cover the changes in pain stimulus, such as those that occur with dressing changes. PCA is commonly used to address the pain of a surgical wound or at the time of a dressing change, particularly a dressing change associated with a burn injury. It is unusual to use PCA within the community/primary care setting and the pain of chronic wounds is better managed by other means. However, PCA is a potential treatment option for patients that have wounds that have been left open to heal by secondary intention while the patient remains in the acute pain phase.

PCA in acute surgical wound pain

PCA is commonly used in the immediate post-operative period

and most surgical nurses will be familiar with the care of patients receiving analgesia in this manner. The type of surgery will not always accurately predict the level of pain expected and, given that pain is subjective, each and every individual will have a varying response to the pain experienced (MacLellan, 2006, *p. 133*). Acute surgical wound pain is described by Kazanowski and Laccetti (2002, *p. 63*) as being incisional pain, occurring secondary to impaired skin integrity following a surgical incision and is probably one of the most well-recognised examples of acute pain. All the physiological factors associated with acute pain apply to the pain experienced after surgery. These can include increased heart rate, blood pressure and respiratory rate, with the patient becoming cold and clammy — all typical of the severe effect on the body of an episode of acute pain. The advent of PCA saw an improvement in the management of acute post-operative pain and followed on from the introduction of acute pain teams into all hospitals where surgery was performed (Royal College of Surgeons of England and the College of Anaesthetists, 1990), allowing the safe introduction and management of this innovative form of analgesic delivery.

Although the analgesia used for PCA can differ according to medical preference and local protocols, the principle behind the use of PCA remains the same.

PCA in burn patients undergoing dressing change

Most people will have experienced a minor burn injury at some time in their life, whether from touching something hot, scalding themselves, or through inadvertently touching a naked flame. The degree of the burn injury is defined by its size and thickness, but there is no doubt that whatever the size or depth, a burn will cause pain (*Chapter 7*). Most people will remember the feeling of a minor burn injury, from the initial (ouch!) phase, to the stinging sensation as the burn is cooled under cold running water, on to the dull background pain that persists through the healing period until eventually the tissues heal and the pain disappears. Severe burns, however, bring additional problems for the patient. The patient will not just experience the pain of the burn injury, but will also have the additional pain of any treatments necessary, such as dressing changes and possible surgery (Barreiro *et al*, 2005).

The initial phase of management of a severe burn injury will require the administration of an opioid analgesic (Drugs and Therapy Perspectives, 2001). Pain management of severe burns in specialist burn units allows for close supervision to enable these patients to have continuous infusion of high dose opioids when appropriate. The acute phase follows the initial phase and lasts until partial-thickness wounds are healed or full-thickness wounds have been grafted (Thomas, 1997, *p. 151*). It is during this phase that background pain becomes a major feature. This pain can be managed by regular analgesia and may become 'low to moderate'. During dressing procedures, however, the pain may become 'severe to excruciating', and it is in the management of this procedural pain that PCA can be of great benefit (Thomas and Rose, 1993). The pain experience of patients with burns usually involves two separate pain components: the constant background pain and the superimposed acute pain experienced during dressing changes or physiotherapy (Sim *et al*, 1996).

The main advantages of using PCA for patients with burns is that the continuous infusion facility can be utilised to treat the background pain, with the demand PCA facility allowing the patient to deliver extra analgesia as and when needed. Before starting a dressing change, a loading dose may be given to allow for the sudden increase in pain from background to acute. Loading patients in this way and using PCA for sudden increases in pain may cause potential sedation and decreased respiratory effort once the dressing has been completed. To lessen these risks, the choice of opioid used is important. Linneman *et al* (2000) advocate the use of fentanyl, as it is of rapid onset, a potent analgesia and short-acting, therefore appropriate for the acute, severe and short duration pain of dressing procedures in burn patients. Following dressing changes patients should be monitored closely for signs of respiratory depression (Sim *et al*, 1996).

Carr and Mann (2000, *p. 160*) suggest that the anxiety associated with burn dressing changes will increase intraprocedure or post-procedure pain. Involving patients in their dressing changes can help to reduce such anxieties (Carr and Mann, 2000). Other strategies include:

- providing information about the intended procedure
- accurately assessing the pain with the patient before, during and after the procedure
- managing the procedure appropriately
- ensuring that the patient has privacy and support throughout the procedure (Kazanowski and Laccetti, 2002, *p. 54*).

Conclusion

Nurses have a pivotal role in the accurate assessment and safe management of patients receiving PCA for acute pain. Nurses initiating PCA should have a sound knowledge and understanding of the mode of delivery, the analgesia, including its properties and side-effects, and have high level pain assessment skills (beginning with believing the patient). Active listening to a patient's pain story will give nurses a wealth of information, which they can use to inform their assessment of the patient's pain and its subsequent management.

References

Barreiro JG, Rodriguez A, Cal M, Alvarez A, Villar FM (2005) Treatment of postoperative pain for burn patients with intravenous analgesia in continuous perfusion using elastomeric infusors. _Burns_ **31**: 67–71

Bhattacharya S, Wang T, Knox F (2006) Analgesia for labour pain-analysis of the trends and associations in the Grampian region of Scotland between 1986 and 2001. _BMC Pregnancy and Childbirth_ **6**: 14

British National Formulary (2008) British National Formulary: 55. BMJ Group and RPS Publishing, London

Boonmak P, Boonmak S, Bunsaengjaroen P, Srichaipanha S, Poomsawat S, Nonlhaopol D (2007) Antiemetic effect of ondansetron 0.2mg mL-1 in PCA morphine solution. _Eur J Anaesthesiol_ **24**(8): 664–7

Bruckenthal P, D'Arcy YM (2007) Assessment and management of pain in older adults: a review of the basics. _Top Adv Nurs Practice_ **7**(1): 8

Carr EC, Mann EM (2000) _Pain Creative Approaches to Effective Management_. Macmillan Press Ltd, London: 2

Carter Snell C, Fothergill-Bourbonnais F, Durovher-Hendriks S (1997) Patient-controlled analgesia and intramuscular injections: a comparison of patient pain experiences and postoperative outcomes. _J Adv Nurs_ **25**: 681–90

Clarke K (1999) Effective pain relief with intrapleural analgesia. _Nurs Times_ **95**(12): 49–50

Clarke K, Iphofen R (2005) Believing the patient with chronic pain: a review of the literature. _Br J Nurs_ **14**(9): 490–3

Clarke K, Iphofen R (2008) Effects of failing to believe patients' experiences of pain. _Nurs Times_ **104**(8): 30–1

Drugs and Therapy Perspectives (2001) Different strategies are needed to manage severe background and procedural burn pain. _Drug and Therapy Perspectives_ **17**(20): 5–8

Evans A (2003) Use of Entonox in the community for control of procedural pain. *Br J Community Nurs* 8(11): 488–94

Hall D (2007) Evaluation of 3 pain assessment tools for use with critically ill adult patients. *Am J Crit Care* 16(3): 309–10

International Association for the Study of Pain (1994) *Classification of Chronic Pain.* IASP Press, Seattle:

International Association for the Study of Pain (1979) *Pain Terms: a list with definitions and notes on usage.* Pain 6: 249–52

Kazanowski MK, Laccetti MS (2002) *Pain.* SLACK Incorporated, New Jersey

Koh P, Thomas VJ (1994) Patient-controlled analgesia (PCA): does time saved by nursing staff improve patient satisfaction with nursing care? *J Adv Nurs* 20: 61–70

Kontrimaviciute E, Baublys A, Ivaskevicius J (2005) Postoperative nausea and vomiting in patients undergoing total abdominal hysterectomy under spinal anaesthesia: a randomized study of ondansetron prophylaxis. *Eur J Anaesthesiol* 22(7): 504–9

Lehman K (2005) Recent developments in patient-controlled analgesia. *J Pain Symptom Management* 29(5S): 72–89

Linneman PK, Terry BE, Burd RS (2000) The efficacy and safety of fentanyl for the management of severe procedural pain in patients with burn injuries. *J Burn Care Rehabilitation* 21(6): 519–22

MacLellan K (2006) *Management of Pain.* Nelson Thornes Ltd, Cheltenham: 3, 65

Macintyre PE, Ready LB (1996) *Acute Pain Management: A Practical Guide.* W B Saunders Company Ltd, London

McDonald AJ, Cooper MG (2001) Patient-controlled analgesia: an appropriate method of pain control in children. *Paediatr Drugs* 3(4): 273–84

Moore A, Edwards J, Barden J, McQuay H (2003) *Bandolier's Little Book of Pain.* Oxford University Press, Oxford: 7

Platt AF Jr, Byrnes JF Jr (2006) Pain assessment tools: guide for healthcare professionals. *Patient Care for the Nurse Pract* July 31

Plaisance L, Logan C (2006) Nursing students' knowledge and attitudes regarding pain. *Pain Management Nurs* 7(4): 167–75

Polomano RC, Rathmell JP, Krenzischek DA, Dunwoody CJ (2008) Emerging trends and new approaches to acute pain management. *Pain Management Nurs* 9(1): S33–S41

Royal College of Surgeons of England and the College of Anaesthetists (1990) *Report of the Working Party on Pain After Surgery.* Royal College of Surgeons of England and the College of Anaesthetists, London

Salmon P, Manyande A (1996) Good patients cope with their pain: post-

operative analgesia and nurses' perceptions of their patients' pain. *Pain*
68: 63–8

Seers K, Friedli K (1996) The patients' experience of their chronic non-malignant pain. *J Adv Nurs* **24**: 1160–8

Shade P (1992) Patient-controlled analgesia: can client education improve outcomes? *J Adv Nurs* **17**: 408–13

Shelley K, Paech MJ (2008) The clinical applications of intranasal opioids. *Curr Drug Delivery* **5**(1): 55–8

Sidebotham D, Schug SA (1997) The safety and utilization of patient-controlled analgesia. *J Pain Symptom Management* **14**(4): 202–9

Sim KM, Hwang NC, Chan YW, Seah CS (1996) Use of patient-controlled analgesia with alfentanil for burns dressing procedures: a preliminary report of five patients. *Burns* **22**(3): 238–41

Smith A, Friedemann ML (1999) Perceived family dynamics of persons with chronic pain. *J Adv Nurs* **30**(3): 543–51

Sofaer B, Walker J (1994) Mood assessment in chronic pain patients. *Disabil Rehab* **16**(1): 35–8

Tarcatu D, Tamasdan C, Moryl N, Obbens E (2007) Are we still scratching the surface? A case of intractable pruritus following systemic opioid analgesia. *J Opioid Management* **3**(3): 167–70

Thomas VJ, Rose FD (1993) Patient-controlled analgesia: a new method for old. *J Adv Nurs* **18**: 1719–26

Thomas VN (1997) *Pain: Its Nature and Management.* Baillière Tindall, London

Viscusi ER (2008) Patient-controlled drug delivery for acute postoperative pain management: a review of current and emerging technologies. *Regional Anaesth Pain Med* **33**(2): 146–58

Walder B, Schafer M, Henzi I, Tramer MR (2001) Efficacy and safety of patient-controlled opioid analgesia for acute postoperative pain. *Acta Anaesthesiol Scand* **45**: 795–804

Waterhouse M (1996) Why pain assessment must start with believing the patient. *Nurs Times* **93**(38): 42

World Union of Wound Healing Societies (2007) Principles of best practice: Minimising pain at wound dressing-related procedures. A consensus document. Toronto, Ontario, Canada: ©WoundPedia Inc

CHAPTER 11

PSYCHOLOGICAL FACTORS OF PAIN PERCEPTION, COMMUNICATION AND RESPONSES TO TREATMENT

Victoria Mason

In 1664 Descartes (cited in Melzack and Wall, 1965) asserted that there was a direct linear relationship between the extent of a person's injury and his or her perception of pain. This widely held view was not seriously challenged until the 1960s, which saw the dawning of a new era in understanding the psychology of pain. This began with the work of Melzack and Wall (1962, 1965), who developed a theory for understanding pain mechanisms that reflected the multifactorial nature of the influences on our perception of pain. A knowledge of these complex influences is important for achieving an understanding of the psychological factors involved in responding to wound pain, how psychological factors might play a part in wound healing itself and how psychological dimensions fit within a more holistic framework of the impact that wound pain has on a person's quality of life.

What is pain?

In the acute phase and during treatment of a wound one of the most salient and attention-grabbing features is the pain associated with the injury itself. Underpinning this, a complex set of reactions is elicited including physiological, immunological, behavioural and emotional responses. There is also a cognitive dimension where a person attaches meaning and significance to the wound in relation to its cause, its appearance and the potential consequences.

According to the International Association for the Study of Pain (IASP), pain is defined as:

*... an unpleasant sensory and emotional experience associated
with actual or potential tissue damage, or described in terms of
such damage (IASP Task Force on Taxonomy, 1994).*

This definition is important because it recognises that pain is not
merely a sensory experience, but that it is accompanied by emotion.
Furthermore, although pain might be the consequence of damaged
tissue, the experience of pain might not be linked to this in a linear way;
equivalent amounts of tissue damage will be experienced differently by
different individuals and the extent of suffering associated with pain
will also vary. This definition also recognises the role that language
plays in communicating pain; while we can never know somebody
else's physical pain, observing non-verbal and verbal behaviour
provides a glimpse of what that person might be experiencing and
enables us to respond appropriately. Indeed, *Principles of Best Practice:
Minimising pain at dressing-related procedures* (World Union of Healing
Societies Initiative, 2007) highlights the importance of observing
non-verbal signs and listening to what the patient is communicating,
reflecting the way in which this definition has been applied in practice.
This definition is not without its detractors, however, as use of the
word 'unpleasant' has been criticised for failing to capture the misery
of pain (Melzack and Wall, 1996).

Models of pain — from Cartesian dualism to the gate control theory

The IASP definition of pain (IASP Task Force on Taxonomy, 1994)
is representative of a broad and ongoing shift away from the
biomedical model, which focuses on biological factors alone, to
a reconceptualisation of pain so that psychosocial factors may be
accounted for.

During the seventeenth century, Descartes proposed that pain was
the result of the pulling on tiny threads at the site of injury, which
was transmitted via nerve impulses direct to a pain centre located in
the brain (Descartes, 1664, cited in Melzack and Wall, 1965). This
was the so-called specificity theory, where pain was believed to be the
direct consequence of sensory input and was proportional to injury.
Later, a number of theories, collectively known as 'pattern theory' were
postulated, where it was proposed that pain impulses were transmitted
to the brain via a pattern of nerve impulses (e.g. Goldscheider, 1894;

Livingston, 1943; Noordenbos, 1959). These early theories were criticised for implying a one-to-one relationship between site and extent of injury, and the intensity of the pain experienced. However, they were consistent with the idea that, like stress, pain primes a person to escape to safety so that recovery from injury can occur. Indeed, this is an adaptive response without which we would be in danger of doing further damage. In the case of chronic pain, however, pain can be experienced or amplified in the absence of nociceptive input because of the plasticity of the central nervous system. These theories, therefore, fail to explain how pain can be maintained when an injury or damage has healed and why, in the context of prolonged pain, the experience of pain may not act as a warning signal.

A number of observations provided mounting evidence that these early theories were not adequate in explaining the pain reported by individuals following injury. Henry Beecher (1959) found that soldiers reported little pain and no need for analgesic medication following quite extensive injuries during battle in the Second World War. In his study comprising a matched group of civilians with similar injuries, Beecher found that the civilians reported considerable pain and the need for medicinal pain relief. Beecher argued that the reported pain was mediated by the meaning it held for the individuals and the context in which the injury occurred: for the injured soldiers, the injury meant that they would be returning home to safety and that they had survived; conversely, the injury experienced by civilians could lead to disability or other potentially negative consequences. Thus, Beecher's observations suggested that reports of pain do not correlate with extent of injury.

Further evidence that pain is not simply proportional to an objectively measurable stimulus comes from studies showing that pain can occur in the absence of damaged tissue, for example in the case of phantom limb pain in amputees (Chahine and Kanazi, 2007), and that, once healed, neuromata at the site of an amputation can continue to be painful (Geraghty and Jones, 1996). In addition, there is extensive evidence for the role of the placebo effect in reducing pain intensity in the absence of any active pharmacological agents (Benedetti, 2006), suggesting that pain is not simply related to the extent of underlying tissue damage.

The principal assumption underpinning the early theories of pain was that the human brain is a passive receiver of stimuli that merely responds to afferent nerve impulses. Given the work of Beecher and the many observations suggesting that this was not the case, Ronald

Melzack, a Canadian psychologist, and a British neuroscientist, Patrick Wall, developed the gate control theory (GCT) of pain from their research attempting to elucidate the mechanisms of pain transmission (Melzack and Wall, 1965) (*Chapter 1*). The GCT provides a powerful metaphor for understanding pain. The hypothetical gate is located in the dorsal horn of the spinal cord and opens and closes in response to information coming in from the periphery (afferent) and from descending (efferent) impulses from the brain. Thus, the brain is no longer the passive receiver of messages, but actively responds to incoming signals and shapes the information sent from the spinal cord to the brain by inhibiting (closing the gate) or exciting cells (opening the gate) surrounding the gating mechanism. If, for example, an individual is in a relaxed and calm state, this may have an inhibitory effect that closes the gate and decreases the perception of pain. Conversely, if a person is highly anxious, this may have the opposite effect of opening the gate and increasing the perception of pain intensity.

Nociceptive information (sensation perceived as painful) is carried by two types of nerve fibre: small-diameter, myelinated A-fibres; and unmyelinated C-fibres. Non-nociceptive (or non-painful) information is carried by large A-beta (A-β) nerve fibres. If the amount of input is greater in these large fibres, this inhibits the amount of information sent to the brain so that less pain is experienced. A classic example of this is when a child hurts him- or herself and the mother rubs it better. In this situation, the large A-β fibres are being stimulated, which closes the gate and the child feels less pain. It must of course be acknowledged that there is a psychosocial dimension to this as well, where the child receives attention and feels cared for, which may also play a role in reducing pain intensity.

There have been some notable criticisms of this theory (Nathan, 1976) and inconsistent empirical evidence. However, its contribution to our understanding of pain mechanisms has had powerful implications for the study, treatment and management of a range of painful conditions and has led to the ascendance of the role of psychological factors in understanding pain. The response to a wound and the intensity of pain experienced varies considerably between individuals, and the GCT provides a framework for understanding the role of cognitive and emotional factors. These include the meaning of the injury, its perceived cause, the role of fear and anxiety in influencing the way an individual responds to the injury creating the wound itself, and the often painful aspects of treatment, such as dressing changes; this latter issue is sometimes referred to as iatrogenic pain (Krasner,

1995). An anxious patient may experience more discomfort than a relaxed one, which means that the relationship between injury and reported pain perception is not a linear or proportionate one, but is influenced by a range of physiological and psychological factors.

The GCT is also consistent with broader developments within health, particularly with the biopsychosocial model that encompasses the role of biological, psychological and social factors in understanding health. The biopsychosocial model was proposed by Engel (1977, 1980), who mounted a long-overdue attack on the biomedical model as its narrow focus excluded some of the important variables shown to influence the experience of pain. Both specificity and pattern theories fitted with the biomedical model's emphasis on physiological factors determining the response to a wound. The biopsychosocial model has been applied to understanding pain (e.g. Gatchel *et al*, 2007; Wiechman Askay and Patterson, 2008), so that biological (extent of wound, activation of small-diameter, myelinated A-nerve fibres and unmyelinated C-nerve fibres), psychological (anxiety, fear) and social (the context in which the injury occurs; the response of other people) factors all mediate the pain experience.

Although the biopsychosocial model has been in the ascendance since the 1970s and has countered some of the inadequacies of the biomedical model, the medical literature tends to focus on its underlying physiological mechanisms. Consequently, the biopsychosocial model has been slow in filtering through to some specialties. Additionally, although the biopsychosocial model is grounded in providing a framework for understanding the response of individuals to injury or harm, it does not help us to understand how biological and psychological factors interact; it merely provides us with different levels of explanation (Cooper *et al*, 1996). However, since the introduction of the GCT and the biopsychosocial model, pain clinicians, anaesthetists, nurses and other healthcare professionals have begun to address the role of psychological factors. This is evidenced by the multidisciplinarity of pain management, particularly chronic pain management, and the acknowledgement of the importance of psychosocial factors in clinical guidelines.

How pain is communicated — behaviour, language and measurement

Pain is communicated in a variety of ways: for example, we can infer it from the extent of the wound or injury; we can observe non-verbal behaviour (wincing, guarded movement, use of medical aids); and we can know of a person's pain from the way he or she talks about it. Of course, it is not always possible to describe pain, and infants and those with intellectual disabilities are unable to convey this in language.

Research in the 1970s reflected a shift towards seeing pain as multidimensional and focused on the language of pain (Melzack and Torgerson, 1971). Given the inherent subjectivity of pain, this had important implications for measurement. Melzack and Torgerson (1971) derived a list of adjectives that were commonly used to describe pain, which led to the development of the McGill Pain Questionnaire (MPQ; Melzack, 1975) that was later abbreviated (Melzack, 1987). The MPQ divided words into:

- those that describe the sensory qualities of pain (e.g. sore)
- those that describe the affective or emotional dimensions (e.g. exhausting)
- those that say something about one's overall assessment or evaluation of the pain (e.g. excruciating)
- those that express its temporal properties (e.g. constant).

The MPQ has been translated into many languages (Yakut *et al*, 2007) and has been shown to be reliable and valid when used clinically (Melzack and Katz, 1992).

There are of course a range of other scales, including visual analogue and numerical rating scales (VAS and NRS respectively; see Lund *et al*, 2005; WUWHS, 2007), and care should be taken in using the most appropriate tools when conducting a thorough assessment of pain.

The language of pain also has a diagnostic value in terms of the way patients use language to describe their pain. The adjectives used describe pain of nociceptive (from tissue damage) or neuropathic (from nerve damage) origin, and provide a clue as to which is the presenting problem. For example, words such as 'aching' and 'throbbing' are associated with pains of nociceptive origin (Ferrante, 1998), while 'burning' and 'shooting' are more generally used when describing neuropathic pain (Gatchel *et al*, 2007). In a study examining the diagnostic value of adjectives in patients with neuropathic pain in France, Boureau *et al* (1990) found that certain adjectives do have a discriminating function for people with different types of pain, and that an adjective list could correctly identify 66% of cases of patients with neuropathic pain.

In addition to specific language used to describe pain, people may also use paralinguistic vocalisations such as moaning, sighing and screaming (Craig and Prkachin, 1983; Skevington, 1995). However, it is not only the verbal behaviour of individuals that communicates pain to others, but also some of the non-verbal signs highlighted above reveal the social nature of the private pain experience. Although much research has examined the role of behavioural manifestations of pain, a particularly interesting avenue has been the investigation of facial expression. For example, there is evidence to suggest that the facial expression of pain is unique and distinct from the way in which the basic emotions are expressed (Craig and Patrick, 1985; Simon *et al*, 2008). Such facial expressions reflect both a response to pain and a social communicative function. An experimental study showed that there are considerable individual differences in the ability of people to accurately distinguish between the facial expressions of people with genuine and faked pain (Hill and Craig, 2004). In a naturalistic context, however, the extent to which these expressions are consciously mediated may be disputed, as may the possible origins of such expressions. However, recognising these expressions in others is part of the complex social dimension of the psychology of wound pain.

A discussion of language, measurement and the expression of pain would not be complete without a consideration of methodological approaches to understanding the psychology of wound pain. This ranges from traditional, positivist, empirical research (such as laboratory experiments and cross-sectional and longitudinal surveys using validated questionnaires or instruments) to more interpretative approaches (e.g. using qualitative methods underpinned by phenomenological or social constructivist principles). Although these yield somewhat different data, both illuminate the role of psychology in wound pain.

The literature using traditional approaches is vast; however, the application of interpretative methodologies to understanding wound pain specifically is somewhat limited. Noticeable exceptions are the use of such approaches to elucidate the views of healthcare professionals toward the care of their patients. For example, Haram *et al* (2003) found that nurses believed that their knowledge on treating wounds was limited, suggesting a need for further training. Kohr and Gibson (2008) highlighted the importance of the therapeutic relationship between patient and caregiver because of the intimacy associated with caring for the patient, including changing dressings. In a study to understand patients' perspectives of the care they receive, Haram and

Dagfinn (2003) found some ambivalence in their views. While patients expressed confidence in the care they received, they simultaneously expressed misgivings about the nature and manner with which the care was carried out. Although these in-depth studies were small in scale, they highlight some of the pertinent issues that patients face when being cared for. They also help healthcare professionals to understand patients' perspectives of their experiences, including the range of psychological factors that influence and are influenced by living with wound pain. However, they tell us little about the pain itself, although this is not surprising given the difficulty of separating this out from other aspects of living with wounds.

Psychological factors of pain perception and pain management

A range of interacting factors play a role and contribute to our understanding of the psychology of wound pain. Eccleston (2001) argues persuasively for the role of psychology in managing pain by identifying some of the key factors that should be considered when treating patients with painful conditions. More broadly, there are a range of so-called basic emotions such as sadness, anger and fear (Ekman, 1992), cognitive factors such as attention, concentration, coping and memory, and social factors including the context within which pain or pain-relieving treatment is delivered, relationship with healthcare professionals and role of spouse, family or significant other. There is also pain behaviour, which signals to others that a person is in pain, and there are attributes of the individuals, such as their age, gender and ethnicity, which may impact on this in light of experience and sociocultural expectations. In addition to the impact of these sociocultural dimensions on the pain experience itself, Dobson (2000) also described the impact of pain on a person's personal and social relationships, highlighting the bi-directional nature of the relationship between an individual with pain and his or her social and cultural context.

In relation to pain and its management, the role of fear has been investigated extensively, particularly in musculoskeletal pain (Leeuw, 2007). In the context of acute injury, fear is an adaptive response to prime the individual to escape and seek help. In chronic pain, however, fear can be dysfunctional and can lead to avoidance behaviour and possible fear of movement (or kinesiophobia), which can lead to functional limitation and increased disability; this is known as fear–avoidance (Vlaeyen and Linton, 2000). Anger is often concomitant with chronic pain (Wade *et al*, 1990; Mason *et al*, 2004), and low mood, sadness or depression may be a response to living with chronic wounds, in addition to fatigue (Price *et al*, 2007). Consequently, identifying and managing anxiety in relation to the distress of painful wound dressing changes is imperative. Although these consequences are far from inevitable, healthcare professionals involved in treating and managing wound pain should at least be aware of the possibility of this range of potential sequelae.

The role of attention and distraction from pain has an important place in the psychology of wound pain and underscores the importance of individual differences. Some individuals derive benefit and are able to distract from nociceptive input, while others are able to attend to and reinterpret the sensations they are experiencing to try and reduce its overall intensity. Such observations have led to the development of a range of distraction techniques, such as immersive virtual reality for burn pain (Hoffman *et al*, 2008) and relaxation for helping patients to manage their pain during wound care (de Jong and Gamel, 2006). Memories and the emotions associated with a previously painful experience also play a role in making sense of and interpreting a person's current situation (Skevington, 1995).

In terms of its common usage, coping with pain refers to how well a person is managing. Within the literature, however, coping refers to a range of strategies that are available to individuals who are faced with a change in health status. Although the range of strategies available is extensive, they can be broadly categorised into approach and avoidance coping strategies (Roth and Cohen, 1986) or problem- and emotion-focused coping strategies (Folkman and Lazarus, 1980):

- *Approach coping* would be directed at the pain, e.g. seeking information to help manage it.
- *Avoidance coping* would involve directing energy into avoiding or ignoring the pain.
- *Problem-focused coping* would involve making attempts to ameliorate the pain with appropriate treatment, making a specific plan and taking responsibility for engaging in self-management.
- *Emotion-focused coping* would include reinterpreting the situation or attempting to regulate the emotional response to the painful wound.

Although it is often assumed that approach and problem-focused coping are more adaptive, people may use different strategies at different times, and healthcare professionals should be sensitive to this.

The context within which the wound occurs and the context of treatment is also crucial to understanding an individual's response, as a wound does not occur in isolation, i.e. it is visible. Although this might appear obvious, it is different from other types of pain that may be invisible, such as musculoskeletal pain. It is important not to focus solely on the wound, but to consider the person to whom the wound has been inflicted. The behaviour of others can be important in understanding the beliefs, attitudes and emotions of the patient, and this should not be forgotten in treating patients with wounds. A patient's interaction with healthcare professionals and the support or otherwise of family or friends may also play a role in how adherent a patient is to his or her self-care regimen. Indeed, it has been suggested that the more congruent the attitudes and beliefs of the patient and heathcare professional, the more likely the patient is to feel motivated to adhere (Cameron, 1996; Jahng *et al*, 2004; Cvengros *et al*, 2007). Moreover, theories such as Health Locus of Control (HLoC; Wallston and Wallston, 1982) shed light on whether a patient feels that he or she (internal), powerful others or chance (external) is most important in recovery or healing. Not surprisingly, patients with a strong internal HLoC are more inclined to engage in self-management, whereas those who have an external HLoC, where they believe that their nurse or doctor should manage and treat their pain, are less likely to engage in this. Data to confirm this are equivocal because there are a multitude of factors influencing the response to treatment. Nonetheless, patient beliefs and the complexity of the treatment milieu play a part in understanding the response to wound pain.

In order to examine the social nature of pain, we can look at the theoretical contribution that psychologists have made to understanding behaviour through consideration of the way that it is influenced by the presence and behaviour of others. For example, despite its chequered history, behaviourism has been applied to understanding a person's response to pain. According to the theory of operant conditioning, behaviour is contingent on rewards and it is argued that so-called pain behaviour (such as wincing and grimacing) is perpetuated because it is rewarded by the attention one receives from others in response to it (Fordyce, 1982). Although it makes intuitive sense, it tends to demonise the patient and has negative connotations through its implication that the patient is consciously and intentionally seeking attention. In reality, a patient is arguably responding quite naturally to the discomfort of pain by displaying this to others verbally and non-verbally. Professionals should be mindful of respecting an individual's verbal and non-verbal expression of pain, while taking care not to reinforce any exaggerated or unnecessary behaviour, although such a distinction is not easy in practice.

A complex set of interacting factors influence the perception of pain and the response to intervention to relieve or enhance the management of pain. In addition to those factors discussed above, underlying physiological processes, such as slower wound healing in the elderly, the meanings that people attach to their experience and the role of culture in defining appropriate displays of pain or discomfort, all play a role in the treatment milieu. The specific influence of gender, age and ethnicity has been examined elsewhere (Skevington, 1995; Berkley, 1997; Fillingim, 2000; Greenspan *et al*, 2007).

The role of psychological factors in wound healing

It is clear that psychological factors impact on the perception and expression of pain. However, psychological factors have also been shown to have a role in wound healing itself. Such research has taken place within the field of psycho-neuro-immunology, which is the study of the relationship between psychological factors, immune functioning and health. Laboratory studies have used punch biopsies as a way to investigate wound healing. One of the major contributions to this area has been the work of Janice Kiecolt-Glaser and colleagues who, using this methodology, found that wound healing was slower among those caring for people with Alzheimer's disease than a control group, suggesting that the stress of care-giving delays healing (Kiecolt-Glaser *et al*, 1995). In a further study, the stress of exams was also shown to delay healing in students (Marucha *et al*, 1998). Although conducted in an experimental setting, these studies show the role of naturalistic acute and chronic stressors on wound healing.

In a recent review, Vileikyte (2007) highlights lacunae in this area in the need for studies on chronic wounds, as much of the research to date has explored the impact of stress on acute wounds. However, it may also be important to consider the temporal nature of the stressor as acute and chronic stress may have different implications for chronic wounds. Elucidating the psychological factors that speed up or delay wound healing would enable the development of interventions to address such factors to promote shorter healing periods and to identify those at risk from delayed healing and its potential consequences.

A challenge to managing wounds is that it involves not only the pain associated with the wound itself, but also iatrogenic factors, such as dressing changes or other procedural aspects of treatment, which may bring about psychological distress and be considered as acutely stressful. Therefore, priority should be given to minimising wound pain to prevent distress and the subsequent delay in healing that such distress may bring about (Soon and Acton, 2006). Careful attention should be paid to treating pain associated with wounds and being sensitive to a patient's response. This is paramount to minimise pain-related distress, while remembering that it is not only pain that generates distress, but also other factors such as the appearance of the wound, its odour, fear of infection or other cognitive or emotional sequelae.

Which psychological outcomes should we be measuring?

Although psychological factors play a key role in understanding the role of pain in wounds, these should not be seen in isolation. Physiological, social and environmental influences constantly interact, influence and are influenced by such processes. Indeed, the essence of the biopsychosocial model is that all these factors should be considered. People with pain do not necessarily see their pain in isolation from other dimensions of their life. Physical comfort is an aspect of quality of life, and a factor that impacts on assessment of life quality. A broader perspective could be advocated, which sees the individual and his or her pain as part of a wider context.

If pain and the associated sensory, affective and cognitive dimensions are to be seen as something impinging on quality of life, in measurement terms the dimensions of pain can be seen as independent or predictor variables, where they predict psychological response and broader outcomes such as quality of life. Conversely, pain and its dimensions can be seen as dependant variables or outcomes themselves, where psychological factors predict reports of pain. The same can be applied to psychological factors themselves; they can be seen as outcomes or predictors of outcome. This highlights the need to assess the pain itself with established rating scales (including the MPQ and VAS) and to assess the impact of pain on functioning (e.g. with the 36-item, short-form health survey (SF-36); Ware and Sherbourne, 1992), and more broadly on quality of life (e.g. with profiles such as the WHOQOL; Skevington, 1999, or indices that calculate a total score). All these measures, including ratings of pain itself, are highly subjective and vulnerable to the same set of response biases that pertain to all psychological measurements. This is not, however, sufficient to override the importance of eliciting this information and is paramount to implementing best practice in managing wounds; patients should feel that their pain is being taken seriously and that it is not being trivialised or dismissed.

Conclusion

This chapter has addressed some of the key issues in understanding the psychology of wound pain, including models of pain, how pain is expressed and communicated, and issues pertaining to its measurement. It has also discussed the factors that influence pain perception and the response to treatment. When a wound occurs it is accompanied by physiological and immunological changes. The person responds to it, attaches meaning to it and experiences an emotional reaction, which is all influenced by previous experience and memories of pain. It happens within a context; in a place and time where it may be witnessed by others who respond accordingly. Pain is inherently subjective and has many dimensions. Psychological factors play a role in the response to treatment and they may themselves delay or promote wound healing.

Research in this area has proliferated in recent decades, and a variety of complementary methodological approaches have been adopted to yield a detailed understanding of a highly subjective and complex human experience. Care should be taken to address some of the psychological factors shown to be important in the experience of pain when managing patients. In addition to understanding the pathophysiological mechanisms of pain, a comprehension of the psychology of wound pain is a core aspect of ensuring that best practice is achieved, which will help ease the suffering of patients and minimise the impact of wound pain on quality of life.

References

Beecher HK (1959) Generalisation from pain of various types and diverse origins. *Science* **130**(3370): 267–8

Benedetti F (2006) Placebo analgesia. *Neurol Sci* **27**(Suppl 2): S100–102

Berkley KJ (1997) Sex differences in pain. *Behav Brain Sci* **20**(3): 371–80; discussion 435–513

Boureau F, Doubrere JF, Luu M (1990) Study of verbal description in neuropathic pain. *Pain* **42**(2): 145–52

Cameron C (1996) Patient compliance: Recognition of factors involved and suggestions for promoting compliance with therapeutic regimens. *J Adv Nurs* **24**(2): 244–50

Chahine L, Kanazi G (2007) Phantom limb syndrome: a review. *Middle East J Anesth* **19**(2): 345–55

Cooper N, Stevenson C, Hale G (1996) The biopsychosocial model. In: Cooper N, C Stevenson C, G Hale G, eds. *Integrating Perspectives on Health*. Open University Press, Buckingham: 1–17

Craig KD, Patrick CJ (1985) Facial expression during induced pain. *J Pers Soc Psychol* **48**(4): 1080–91

Craig KD, Prkachin KM (1983) Non-verbal measures of pain. In: Melzack R, ed. *Pain Measurement and Assessment*. Raven Press, New York: 173–82

Cvengros JA, Christensen AJ, Hillis SL, Rosenthal GE (2007) Patient and physician attitudes in the health care context: Attitudinal symmetry predicts patient satisfaction and adherence. *Ann Behav Med* **33**(3): 262–8

de Jong AE, Gamel C (2006) Use of a simple relaxation technique in burn care: literature review. *J Adv Nurs* **54**(6): 710–21

Descartes R (1664) Cited in: Melzack R, Wall PD (1965) Pain mechanisms: a new theory. *Science* **150**: 971

Dobson F (2000) The art of pain management. *Prof Nurse* **15**(12): 789–90

Eccleston C (2001) Role of psychology in pain management. *Br J Anaesth* **87**(1): 144–52

Ekman P (1992) Are there basic emotions? *Psychol Rev* **99**(3): 550–3

Engel GL (1977) The need for a new medical model: a challenge for biomedicine. *Science:* **196**(4286): 129–36

Engel GL (1980) The clinical application of the biopsychosocial model. *Am J Psychiatry* **137**(5): 535–44

Ferrante FM (1998) The pharmacologic management of chronic orthopaedic pain. *UPOJ* **11**: 73–8

Fillingim RB (2000) Sex, gender, and pain: Women and men really are different. *Curr Rev Pain* **4**(1): 24–30

Folkman S, Lazarus RS (1980) An analysis of coping in a middle-aged community sample. J *Health Social Behav* **21**(3): 219–39

Fordyce WE (1982) A behavioural perspective on chronic pain. *Br J Clin Psychol* **21**(4): 313–20

Gatchel RJ, Peng YB, Peters ML, Fuchs PN, Turk DC (2007) The biopsychosocial approach to chronic pain: scientific advances and future directions. *Psychol Bull* **133**(4): 581–624

Geraghty TJ, Jones LE (1996) Painful neuromata following upper limb amputation. *Prosthet Orthot Int* **20**(3): 176–81

Goldscheider A (1894) *Uber den schmerzs in physiologischer und klinischer hinsicht.* Hirschwald, Berlin

Greenspan JD, Craft RM, LeResche L, Arendt-Nielsen L, Berkley KJ, Fillingim RB, *et al* (2007) Studying sex and gender differences in pain and analgesia: A consensus report. *Pain* **132**(Suppl 1): S26–45

Haram R, Ribu E, Rustoen T (2003) The views of district nurses on their level of knowledge about the treatment of leg and foot ulcers. *J Wound Ostomy Continence Nurs* **30**(1): 25–32

Haram RB, Dagfinn N (2003) Errors and discrepancies: a patient perspective on leg ulcer treatment at home. *J Wound Care* **12**(5): 195–9

Hill ML, Craig KD (2004) Detecting deception in facial expressions of pain: accuracy and training. *Clin J Pain* **20**(6): 415–22

Hoffman HG, Patterson DR, Seibel E, Soltani M, Jewett-Leahy L, Sharar SR (2008) Virtual reality pain control during burn wound debridement in the hydrotank. *Clin J Pain* **24**(4): 299–304

IASP Task Force on Taxonomy (1994) *Classification of Chronic Pain: Descriptions of Chronic Pain Syndromes and Definitions of Pain Terms.* IASP Press, Seattle

Jahng KH, Martin LR, Golin CE, DiMatteo MR (2005) Preferences for medical collaboration: Patient-physician congruence and patient outcomes. *Patient Education Counseling* **57**(3): 308–14

Kiecolt-Glaser JK, Marucha PT, Malarkey WB, Mercado AM, Glaser R (1995) Slowing of wound healing by psychological stress. *Lancet* **346**(8984): 1194–6

Kohr R, Gibson M (2008) Doing the right thing: Using hermeneutic phenomenology to understand management of wound pain. *Ostomy/ Wound Management* **54**(4): 52–60

Krasner D (1995) The chronic wound pain experience. *Ostomy Wound Management* **41**(3): 20–5

Leeuw M, Goossens ME, Linton SJ, Crombez G, Boersma K, Vlaeyen JW (2007) The fear-avoidance model of musculoskeletal pain: Current state of scientific evidence. *J Behav Med* **30**(1): 77–94

Livingston WK (1943) *Main mechanisms*. Macmillan, New York

Lund I, Lundeberg T, Sandberg L, Budh CN, Kowalski J, Svensson E (2005) Lack of interchangeability between visual analogue and verbal rating pain scales: a cross-sectional description of pain etiology groups. *BMC Med Res Methodol* 5: 31

Marucha PT, Kiecolt-Glaser JK, Favagehi M (1998) Mucosal wound healing is impaired by examination stress. *Psychosom Med* 60(3): 362–5

Mason VL, Skevington SM, Osborn M (2004) Development of a pain and discomfort module for use with the WHOQOL-100. *Qual Life Res* 13(6): 1139–52

Melzack R (1975) The McGill Pain Questionnaire: major properties and scoring methods. *Pain* 1(3): 277–99

Melzack R (1987) The short-form McGill Pain Questionnaire. *Pain* 30(2): 191–7

Melzack R, Katz J (1992) The McGill Pain Questionnaire; appraisal and current status. In: Turk DC, Melzack R, eds. *Handbook of Pain Assessment*. Guilford, New York, London

Melzack R, Torgerson WS (1971) On the language of pain. *Anesthesiology* 34(1): 50–9

Melzack R, Wall PD (1962) On the nature of cutaneous sensory mechanisms. *Brain* 85: 331–56

Melzack R, Wall PD (1965) Pain mechanisms: a new theory. *Science*: 150(699): 971–9

Melzack R, Wall PD (1996) *The Challenge of Pain*. 2nd edn. Penguin Books, London

Nathan PW (1976) The gate-control theory of pain. *Brain* 99(1): 123–58

Noordenbos W (1959) *Pain*. Elsevier, Amsterdam:

Simon D, Craig KD, Gosselin F, Belin P, Rainville P (2008) Recognition and discrimination of prototypical dynamic expressions of pain and emotions. *Pain* 135(1-2): 55–64

Skevington SM (1995) *Psychology of Pain*. John Wiley and Sons, Chichester

Skevington SM (1999) Measuring quality of life in Britain: an introduction to the WHOQOL-100. *J Psychosomat Res* 47(5): 449–59

Soon K, Acton C (2006) Pain-induced stress: a barrier to wound healing. *Wounds UK* 2(4): 92–101

Vlaeyen JWS, Linton SJ (2000) Fear-avoidance and its consequences in chronic musculoskeletal pain: a state of the art. *Pain* 85(3): 317–32

Ware JE Jr, Sherbourne CD (1992) The MOS 36-item short-form health survey (SF-36): I. Conceptual framework and item selection. *Med Care* 30: 473–83

Wiechman Askay S, Patterson DR (2008) What are the psychiatric sequelae of burn pain? *Curr Pain Headache Rep* 12(2): 94–7

World Union of Wound Healing Societies (2007) Principles of best practice: Minimising pain at wound dressing-related procedures. A consensus document. Toronto, Ontario, Canada: ©WoundPedia Inc

Yakut Y, Yakut E, Bayar K, Uygur F (2007) Reliability and validity of the Turkish version short-form McGill Pain Questionnaire in patients with rheumatoid arthritis. *Clin Rheumatol* **26**(7): 1083–7

CHAPTER 12

MULTINATIONAL SURVEY OF THE ASSESSMENT OF PAIN WHEN REMOVING DRESSINGS

Richard White

Wounds to the skin, both acute and chronic, can present in a huge variety of forms, affecting all areas of the body and posing different management problems. Generally wounds have to be treated with dressings that will cover and protect them. These dressings often have to be retained in place with retention bandages or tapes so that they do not slip. Alternatively, dressings may have adhesive contact layers as integral components that adhere directly to the wound or adjacent peri-wound skin. These adhesive dressings may present problems when they are removed, as they can cause significant levels of trauma to the wound or adjacent skin, resulting in pain for the patient (Dykes *et al*, 2001; Dykes and Heggie, 2003).

Pain is a significant problem with all types of wounds and the pain that patients experience may be associated with the wounds themselves, dressings or dressing changes. The treatment of pain has been highlighted as an area of concern and focus for healthcare workers.

The World Union of Wound Healing Societies' (WUWHS) consensus document on minimising pain at wound dressing-related procedures recommends that wound-related pain should be assessed and its intensity rated before, during, and after dressing procedures and that practice should be reviewed if pain is rated as moderate or more (for example, a pain score higher than 4 on a scale of 1–10) (WUWHS, 2004). The review of practice should consider current dressing regimens. The highest levels of pain are generally associated with skin and wound damage that occurs during dressing changes (Gerritsen *et al*, 1994; European Wound Management Association [EWMA], 2002; Tokumura *et al*, 2005; Dykes, 2007).

The first step in treating pain is acknowledging that it exists, ascertaining when it occurs and then identifying its primary causes. The most appropriate means for managing the pain and providing supportive measures can then be given. As part of the treatment regimen, routine assessment (at the beginning of and during treatment) should be undertaken. This will enable appropriate changes to be made to treatment regimens that meet the needs of the patient. Assessment tools such as visual analogue scales (VAS) are routinely used to measure levels of pain in patients with wounds (World Union of Wound Healing Societies, 2004; Franks *et al*, 2007). Using such tools, a regimen for relieving pain and stress should be developed for individual patients, for example offering analgesics and/or psychological (*Chapter 11*) and other non-drug therapies (*Chapter 9*), as outlined by Acton (2007) and summarised in *Table 12.1*.

Dressings that use Safetac soft silicone adhesive technology (Mölnlycke Health Care, Gothenberg) have been shown to benefit the patient by minimising the risk of trauma and pain associated with the use of adhesive dressings (White, 2005). Examples of products utilising Safetac technology include:

- Mepilex®, Mepilex® Heel, Mepilex® Lite (absorbent soft silicone foam dressing)
- Mepilex® Ag (antimicrobial soft silicone foam dressing)
- Mepilex® Border, Mepilex® Border Lite/Mepilex® Border Sacrum (self-adherent soft silicone foam dressing)
- Mepilex® Transfer (soft silicone exudate transfer dressing)
- Mepitel® (soft silicone wound contact layer).

To further understand the clinical implications of using these dressings, a multinational clinical survey of patients with a variety of different wound types was undertaken, funded by Mölnlycke Health Care.

Aims

The objective of the survey was to assess the impact of introducing advanced dressings with Safetac soft silicone adhesive technology (dressings with Safetac technology) on levels of wound trauma and pain, compared with a previous regimen of advanced dressings with traditional adhesives (traditional adhesive-based dressings) (for analysis purposes these dressings were categorised into adhesive foams, hydrocolloids and others including films, surgical dressings and alginates).

Table 12.1: Methods of relieving pain in patients with chronic wounds (summarised from Acton, 2007)	
Pharmacological therapies	• Opioid analgesics (fast-acting but adverse effects can be problematic) • Topical anaesthetic agents (doubtful efficacy) • Non-steroidal anti-inflammatory agents (limited supportive data)
Psychological and other non-pharmacological therapies	• Cognitive behavioural therapy (CBT) • Relaxation • Hypnosis • Transcutaneous electrical nerve stimulation (TENS) • Acupuncture • Energy healing • Physical therapy • Distraction (e.g. music) • Guided imagery • Biofeedback • Meditation and prayer
Wound care products	To reduce anxiety associated with dressing-related procedures, appropriate dressings should be selected that: • promote moist wound healing • do not dry out • stay *in situ* for long periods • do not leak • prevent trauma to wounds and surrounding skin* *Soft silicone dressings fulfil these criteria: they have low peel strengths to reduce damage, are designated as atraumatic and can prevent wound trauma

Methods

Patients being treated with a traditional adhesive-based dressing (i.e. a dressing with either a polyurethane, or an acrylic, or a hydrocolloid-based adhesive) as either a primary or secondary dressing were included in the survey. Clinicians who were experienced in the provision of wound care and who were using advanced dressings with traditional-based adhesives as part of their treatment regimen were asked to participate. Patients with chronic and traumatic wounds that were deemed by the clinicians to be suitable were included in the survey. (Patients with infected wounds were excluded.) As this was a survey and not a formal clinical trial, recruitment was done on an ad-hoc basis from the participating countries (*Table 12.2*).

Table 12.2: Participating countries	
Australia	Italy
Austria	Lithuania
Belgium	Netherlands
Czech Republic	Norway
Denmark	Slovenia
Dubai	Spain
Estonia	Sweden
Finland	Taiwan
France	UK
Germany	USA

The patients were asked to record their level of pain before, during and after dressing removal rating the pain on a scale of 0–10 (0 = no pain to 10 = unbearable pain). The VAS has been validated for measuring pain severity in patients with wounds (Freeman *et al*, 2001). It is easy to use and most patients, even with cognitive impairment, are able to use it to indicate their pain severity (Harms-Ringdahl *et al*, 1986). The VAS used in this study is listed as a suitable pain assessment tool in a consensus document produced by the World Union of Wound Healing Societies (2004).

The severity of trauma to the wound and peri-wound skin was also evaluated by a qualitative visual assessment carried out by the investigators, all of whom were instructed to use a standardised assessment form. Patients were then switched to a second treatment regimen involving a dressing with Safetac technology (Mepilex, Mepilex Lite, Mepilex Border, or Mepilex Border Lite). At the next dressing change (visit 2), trauma and pain levels were measured, recorded, and compared with those obtained at visit 1. A statistical analysis on the pain scorres was undertaken using a t-test.

Results

Baseline characteristics

A total of 3034 patients were involved in the survey. Data relating to the age of the participants are presented in *Figure 12.1*. Patients presented with a variety of wound types, including leg ulcers (venous, arterial and mixed aetiologies), burns, skin tears, pressure ulcers and diabetic foot ulcers (*Figure 12.2*). *Figure 12.3* demonstrates the number of different dressings used at baseline, the majority being adhesive foams

($n = 1445$), hydrocolloids ($n = 1095$) and other dressings ($n = 495$) such as films, surgical dressings and alginates.

Evaluation of trauma

Data relating to trauma associated with the traditional adhesive-based dressings at visit 1 compared with that associated with the dressings utilising Safetac technology at visit 2 are presented in *Figure 12.4*. The results at visit 1 demonstrate that about 10% of responses indicated high levels of trauma; 28–39% of the responses indicated moderate levels; 31–35% indicated very slight trauma; and 18–29% indicated no trauma associated with the traditional adhesive-based

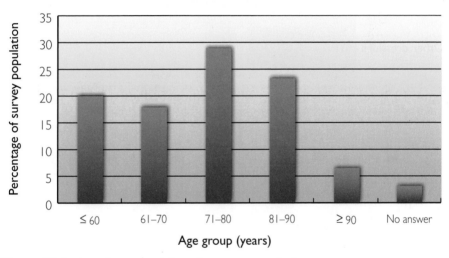

Figure 12.1: Age demographics of survey population

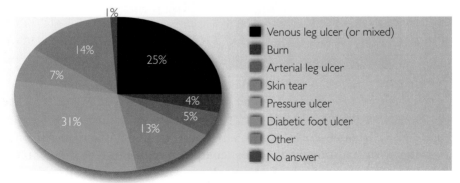

Figure 12.2: Wound types included in the survey

225

dressings. In comparison, the results at visit 2 demonstrate that only 1% of responses indicated high levels of trauma; 11% of the responses indicated moderate levels; 35–37% indicated very slight trauma, and about 50% indicated no trauma associated with the dressings utilising Safetac technology.

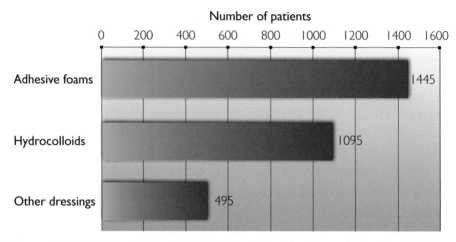

Figure 12.3: Advanced dressings with traditional adhesives used at baseline

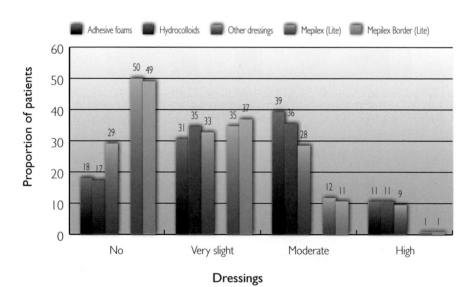

Figure 12.4: Trauma scores at visit 1 (wounds treated with advanced dressings with traditional adhesives) compared with those obtained at visit 2 (wounds treated with foam dressings with Safetac soft silicone adhesive technology)

Evaluation of pain

Data relating to pain (before, during and after dressing removal) associated with the traditional adhesive-based dressings at visit 1 compared with that associated with the dressings utilising Safetac technology at visit 2 are presented in _Figure 12.5._

The results from this study show that at visit 1 the ranges of VAS pain scores reported with the traditional adhesive-based dressings were:

- before removal of the dressings: 2.4–3.2
- at the time of the dressing changes: 4.6–5.2
- after dressing changes: 2.9–3.9.

It was evident that there was a consistent trend associated with all of the traditional adhesive-based dressings evaluated where pain levels increased during their removal.

In comparison, significantly lower pain scores $(p=0.01)$ were reported at visit 2 after the patients had been treated with the dressings utilising Safetac technology compared with those reported at visit 1

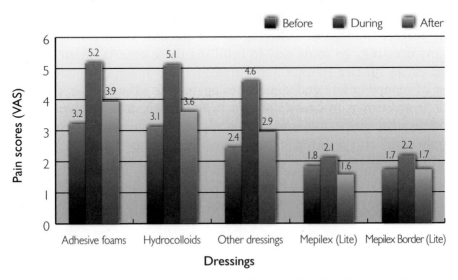

Figure 12.5: Pain scores at visit 1 (wounds treated with advanced dressings with traditional adhesives) compared with those obtained at visit 2 (wounds treated with foam dressings with Safetac soft silicone adhesive technology) before, during and after dressing removal

after the patients had been treated with traditional adhesive-based dressings (*Table 12.3*).

The ranges of VAS pain scores at visit 2 were:

- before removal of the dressings: 1.7–1.8
- at the time of the dressing changes: 2.1–2.2
- after dressing changes: 1.6–1.7.

Unlike the traditional adhesive-based dressings, the dressings with Safetac technology were not associated with increased pain at dressing changes. The pain scores at visit 2 remained low and consistent throughout the dressing changes.

When asked about dressing preference, more than 90% of patients surveyed indicated that they preferred the dressings with Safetac technology to their previous dressing regimen (*Figure 12.6*).

Discussion

There are a number of criteria that have been listed as necessary to create an optimum wound dressing (Dale, 1997; Morgan, 1998). Essentially, a dressing should provide protection for the wound and an optimum environment for healing but, above all, it must not cause any further damage or suffering to the patient. Unfortunately, while many dressings go some way to fulfilling these criteria, many of them can cause further trauma and subsequent pain for the patient. The use of inappropriate and sometimes aggressive adhesives on dressings has been shown to cause damage to the newly forming wound bed and/or adjacent peri-wound skin, and the damage caused by repeated application and removal of adhesive dressings is the main cause of

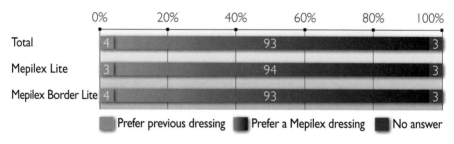

Figure 12.6: Preferred dressing use after completion of survey

trauma to wounds and peri-wound skin (Dykes *et al*, 2001; Dykes and Heggie, 2003; Dykes, 2007).

This trauma can give rise to variable levels of inflammatory skin damage — oedema, soreness and adverse effects on skin barrier function (Gerritsen *et al*, 1994; Dykes and Heggie, 2003; Dykes, 2007). In a series of studies, Dykes has shown that some traditional adhesive-based dressings which use acrylic-based adhesives can be more aggressive than others using Safetac soft silicone adhesive technology. When applied to the skin of volunteers with healthy skin it has been shown that traditional adhesive-based dressings demonstrate a greater degree of damage to the stratum corneum (Dykes *et al*, 2001), higher levels of discomfort (Dykes and Heggie, 2003) and skin damage as measured by transepidermal water loss (TEWL) with greater discomfort measured using a cumulative irritancy score (Dykes, 2007). With the physical trauma caused to the wound and skin, it has been suggested that

Table 12.3: Statistical analysis of pain scores: traditional adhesive-based dressings versus dressings with Safetac technology

Parameter	Average pain scores (VAS) ($n = 3034$)
Before removal: 1st visit (advanced dressings utilising traditional adhesives)	3.0
Before removal: 2nd visit (dressing with Safetac technology)	1.8
Difference	-1.2
Significance	$p = 0.01$
At removal: 1st visit (advanced dressing utilising traditional adhesives)	5.1
At removal: 2nd visit (dressing with Safetac technology)	2.2
Difference	-2.9
Significance	$p = 0.01$
After removal: 1st visit (advanced dressing utilising traditional adhesives)	3.6
After removal: 2nd visit (dressing with Safetac technology)	1.7
Difference	-1.9
Significance	$p = 0.01$

patients suffer stress as a result of pain related to dressings and dressing changes which may, in turn, be detrimental to the healing process (Soon and Acton, 2006; Coulling, 2007; Vileikyte, 2007).

A further problem associated with traditional adhesive-based dressings is pain resulting from the damage that they can cause to wounds and peri-wound skin. Pain is a major problem and is most often related to inappropriate dressing selection. The selection of a suitable, non-adherent dressing which will result in greater patient acceptability is a very important part of the holistic approach to treatment (Meaume et al, 2004).

A number of studies have looked at the impact of pain in patients with a variety of different wounds. In a large study undertaken to evaluate the incidence of pain in 5,850 patients with acute ($n = 2,914$) or chronic wounds ($n = 2,936$) of various causes during dressing removal, and to evaluate the effect of switching to a non-adherent dressing, patients with both types of wounds reported 'moderate to severe' pain during the medical screening visit (79.9% and 79.7%) and 'very severe' pain in their self-evaluation questionnaire completed at home (47% and 59% respectively) (Meaume et al, 2004). Dressing removal was found to be most painful when there was adherence to the wound bed. Switching to a new, non-adherent dressing reduced pain during dressing changes in 88% of patients with chronic wounds and 95% of patients with acute wounds.

A recent one-day survey was undertaken at a university hospital in Paris, France. The purpose of the study was to evaluate the prevalence, clinical aspects and management of wounds in the hospital by undertaking a 'snapshot' survey of all hospitalised patients to ascertain the prevalence of wounds and the provision of wound care on one specific day in April 2005. The results demonstrated that, out of a total of 624 patients examined, 327 (52%) had 933 wounds (an average of 2.8 per patient). Importantly, pain at wound dressing changes was treated in 89% of cases (Mahé et al, 2006). The findings of Mahé et al highlight that pain at wound dressing change is endemic and, furthermore, often requires a treatment intervention, thus emphasising the need for appropriate dressing usage and dressing change procedures.

A recently published article has highlighted the fact that a high percentage (60%) of patients with venous leg ulcers and other types of chronic wounds exhibit pain, the result of which is detrimental to the well-being of patients (Price et al, 2007) and can delay healing (Soon and Acton, 2006). Price et al underline the message that pain and its cause should be handled as one of the main priorities in chronic wound management, that assessment should be undertaken routinely, and if this is not done then it will lead to patient suffering and increased costs to healthcare service providers (Price *et al*, 2007).

Pain associated with trauma can, in some instances, be considerable, notably when dressings are changed, and is a concern in patients with chronic wounds (e.g. venous leg ulcers) and friable peri-wound skin. As a consequence, pain management has become a major part of wound care with many organisations and care providers incorporating the management of wound pain into standards and guidelines. The European Wound Management Association (EWMA) has developed a position document that provides clinical recommendations on how to assess and manage wound pain (EWMA, 2002).

The results from this large multinational clinical survey demonstrate that foam dressings with Safetac soft silicone adhesive, when used in the place of some types of adhesive foams and hydrocolloids, reduce traumatic injuries to the wound or adjacent tissue. The introduction of dressings with Safetac technology resulted in a reduction in the levels of trauma compared with those reported with the advanced dressings utilising traditional adhesive systems. For example, the percentage of responses indicating no trauma with the dressings utilising Safetac technology was almost double that recorded for the advanced dressings with traditional adhesives. The findings also demonstrate that the dressings are associated with clinically significant reductions in levels of wound-associated pain at dressing changes. The low pain scores recorded immediately before dressing change reflect the low levels of pain associated with foam dressings using Safetac soft silicone technology during wear, even though the scores could have been influenced by patients anticipating possible effects of the imminent dressing removals.

The pain scores in this multinational survey seem relatively low when compared with pain scores from patients with wounds reported in the published literature. For example, in a study that was undertaken to evaluate the application of a topical collagen matrix to patients with venous leg ulcers (Wollina *et al*, 2005), one of the objectives was to measure pain associated with the wound. The mean VAS pain scores before treatment were reported to be 8.72 and 7.88, for the treatment and non-treatment groups respectively. After one week of treatment, the scores dropped to 5.76 and 6.66, although the treated group did show a reduction in pain scores to 3.84 in the second week of treatment. Overall the scores were notably higher than seen in the multinational survey presented in this chapter. Another study investigated pain as measured by VAS in patients with skin graft sites treated with three different dressings (Poonyakariyagorn *et al*, 2002). The pain scores associated with two film dressings were comparable to those obtained in this survey, whereas the pain scores associated with a tulle gauze dressing were much higher. The low pain scores may be explained, at least in part, by the fact that the patients reported their pain scores to the investigators who actually undertook the dressing changes, although this practice is in line with the recommendations of the World Union of Wound Healing Societies in relation to pain assessment (WUWHS, 2004).

Pain scores are also related to the wound type: some wounds are more painful than others, and some wounds may present with little or no pain. It might, therefore, be appropriate to group this data according to wound type in order to obtain a more detailed view of the ability of foam dressings with Safetac soft silicone adhesive technology to reduce pain.

Conclusion

Trauma to wounds or peri-wound skin may exacerbate the condition leading to delayed healing or further wound complications. Pain leading to increased stress in patients has also been implicated in contributing to a delayed healing response. In view of this, the use of dressings that do not cause trauma and pain present obvious benefits to patients, as well as clinical benefits by having the potential to shorten healing times which ultimately makes better use of the limited resources available to health workers treating chronic wounds.

The results of this survey demonstrate that dressings that include Safetac soft silicone adhesive technology benefit patients in terms of significantly reducing pain during wear (as indicated by the pain scores recorded immediately before dressing change), at dressing removal, and after dressing change, when compared with advanced dressings that use traditional adhesives.

References

Acton C (2007) The holistic management of chronic wound pain. *Wounds UK* 3(1): 61–9

Coulling S (2007) Fundamentals of pain management in wound care. *Br J Nurs* **16**(13): S4–S12

Dale J (1997) Wound dressings. *Prof Nurse* **12** (Suppl): S12–S14

Dykes PJ (2007) The effect of adhesive dressing edges on cutaneous irritancy and skin barrier function. *J Wound Care* **16**(3): 97–100

Dykes PJ, Heggie R, Hill SA (2001) Effects of adhesive dressings on the stratum corneum of skin. *J Wound Care* **10**(2): 7–10

Dykes PJ, Heggie R (2003) The link between the peel force of adhesive dressings and subjective discomfort in volunteer subjects. *J Wound Care* **12**(7): 260–2

European Wound Management Association (2002) Position Document: *Pain at wound dressing changes*. London: MEP Ltd

Franks PJ, Moody M, Moffatt CJ, *et al* (2007) Randomized trial of two foam dressings in the management of chronic venous ulceration. *Wound Repair Regen* **15**(2): 197–202

Freeman K, Smyth C, Dallam L, Jackson B (2001) Pain measurement scales: a comparison of the visual analogue and faces rating scales in measuring pressure ulcer pain. *J Wound Ostomy Cont Nurs* **28**(6): 290–6

Gerritsen MJ, van Erp PE, van Vlijmen-Willems IM, *et al* (1994) Repeated tape stripping of normal skin: a histological assessment and comparison with events seen in psoriasis. *Arch Dermatol Res* **286**(8): 455–61

Harms-Ringdahl K, Carlsson AM, Ekholm J, Raustorp A, Svensson T, Toresson HG (1986) Pain assessment with different intensity scales in response to loading of joint structures. *Pain* **27**: 401–11

Mahé E, Langlois G, Baron G, *et al* (2006) Results of a comprehensive hospital-based wound survey. *J Wound Care* **15**(9): 381–4

Meaume S, Teot L, Lazareth I, Martini J, Bohbot S (2004) The importance of pain reduction through dressing selection in routine wound management: the MAPP study. *J Wound Care* **13**(10): 409–13

Morgan DA (1998) The application of the 'ideal dressing' theory to practice. *Nursing Scotland* July: 16–8

Poonyakariyagorn T, Sirimaharaj W, Pinchai O, Angspatt A (2002) Comparison among Op-site, polyvinyl chloride film and tulle gauze in the treatment of skin graft donor site. *J Med Assoc Thai* **85**(4): 455–61

Price P, Fogh K, Glynn C, Krasner DL, Osterbrink J, Sibbald RG (2007) Managing painful chronic wounds: the wound pain management model. *Int Wound J* **4**(S1): 4–15

Soon K, Acton C (2006) Pain-induced stress: a barrier to wound healing. *Wounds UK* **2**(4): 92–101

Tokumura F, Umekage K, Sado M, *et al* (2005) Skin irritation due to repetitive application of adhesive tape: the influence of adhesive strength and seasonal variability. *Skin Res Technol* **11**(2): 102–6

Vileikyte L (2007) Stress and wound healing. *Clin Dermatol* **25**(1): 49–55

White R (2005) Evidence for atraumatic soft silicone wound dressing use. *Wounds UK* **1**(3): 104–9

Wollina U, Schmidt WD, Krönert C, Nelskamp C, Scheibe A, Fassler D (2005) Some effects of a topical collagen-based matrix on the microcirculation and wound healing in patients with chronic venous leg ulcers: preliminary observations. *Int J Low Extrem Wounds* **4**(4): 214–24

World Union of Wound Healing Societies (2004) Principles of best practice: Minimising pain at wound dressing-related procedures. A consensus document. London: MEP Ltd. Available online at: www.wuwhs.org/pdf/consensus_eng.pdf [last accessed 20th August, 2007]

INDEX